HOUSTON

including
Huntsville, Beaumont, and Galveston

LAURIE RODDY

MENASHA RIDGE PRESS
Birmingham, Alabama

ISBN 978-0-89732-913-2

Cover by Scott McGrew
Text design by Annie Long
Maps by Laurie Roddy, Scott McGrew, and Chris Erichson
Cover photo by Laurie Roddy
Author photo by Jim Roddy
All other photos by Laurie Roddy

MENASHA RIDGE PRESS
P.O. Box 43673
Birmingham, AL 35243
www.menasharidge.com

DISCLAIMER

This book is meant only as a guide to select trails in the Houston area and does not guarantee hiker safety in any way—you hike at your own risk. Neither Menasha Ridge Press nor Laurie Roddy is liable for property loss or damage, personal injury, or death that result in any way from accessing or hiking the trails described in the following pages. Please be aware that hikers have been injured in the Houston area. Be especially cautious when walking on or near boulders, steep inclines, and drop-offs, and do not attempt to explore terrain that may be beyond your abilities. To help ensure an uneventful hike, please read carefully the introduction to this book, and perhaps get further safety information and guidance from other sources. Familiarize yourself thoroughly with the areas you intend to visit before venturing out. Ask questions, and prepare for the unforeseen. Familiarize yourself with current weather reports, maps of the area you intend to visit, and any relevant park regulations.

Contents

About the Author

Laurie Roddy

A native of Houston, Laurie has been writing for more than 25 years on everything from computers to the outdoors. She started her own company, Roddy Communications, Inc., in 1997 after having worked for 10 years as a technical writer for Compaq Computer Corporation. Her main interests and current writing topics include hiking 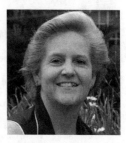 and the outdoors, travel, golf, and nonprofit organizations. She has hiked the Rocky Mountains, Mounts Olympia and Rainier, the Davis Mountains, the Great Smoky Mountains, 60 miles of the Tahoe Rim Trail, Big Bend and Virgin Islands national parks, and all around the Houston area. She is a contributing writer for *Cy-Fair Magazine, Community Impact News* for northwest Houston, and **Trails.com.** Laurie is also the Houston Hiking Examiner for **Examiner.com.**

Introduction

Welcome to *Easy Hikes Close to Home: Houston*. This title in the Easy Hikes series is organized according to three Greater Houston regions: Urban Houston, State Parks near Houston, and Outlying Areas.

Numbered map icons on the inside front cover indicate each primary trailhead and are keyed to the table of contents and narrative text for each trail. On the inside back cover, a map legend defines symbols for parking, restrooms, trail features, and other details. Armed with this handy guidebook, you can quickly head out the door and, well, take a hike!

OVERVIEW

Each hike description starts with a box that gives you the essentials: route mileage and configuration, probable hiking time, and brief notes about scenery, sun exposure, trail access, additional maps, restrooms, and other information. The description ends with driving directions to the trailhead; in some cases, suggestions for nearby activities follow the driving directions. Those with GPS devices can punch in the trailhead coordinates incorporated into each trail map and let their devices guide the way. Mileage shown for each hike corresponds to the total distance, from start to finish, for loops, out-and-backs, and balloon hikes. You can shorten or extend some of these hikes with connecting trails.

TRAIL MAPS

Maps for each hike include GPS coordinates. Based on data downloaded from the author's handheld GPS unit and then plotted onto a digital U.S. Geological Survey (USGS) topographic map, the coordinates are shown as both latitude–longitude as well as UTM (Universal Transverse Mercator) coordinates (WGS84).

HIKING ESSENTIALS

Boots should be your footwear of choice. Sport sandals are popular, but they leave much of your foot exposed and vulnerable to hazardous plants, thorns, rocks, and sharp twigs.

When it comes to water, err on the side of excess. Hydrate prior to your hike, carry (and drink) six ounces of water for every mile you plan to hike, and hydrate after the hike. Pack along a couple of small bottles even for short hikes. You may decide to linger on the trail or take an alternate route and extend your time outdoors.

Always plan for unpredictable scenarios by carrying these items, in addition to water:

Map (*even if you have a GPS device, always bring a map*)

Compass

Basic first-aid supplies, *such as adhesive bandages and aspirin*

Knife

Windproof matches or a lighter and fire starter

Snacks

Flashlight with extra batteries

Rain protection and a sweater or windbreaker, *even in warm weather during the fall or spring*

Sun protection

Insect repellent

Whistle

GENERAL TIPS

The whole point of your hike is to enjoy nature, fresh air, and exercise. Here are a few tips to enhance your excursion:

- Avoid weekends and traditional holidays in the state parks if possible; otherwise, go early in the morning.
- Before you hit the trail, double-check your map, and don't set out on the trail until you have the information you need.

- Once on the trail, watch your step. A sprained ankle can ruin a trip very quickly.

- Hike on open trails only. Respect trail and road closures, avoid trespassing on private land, and obtain permits if required. Leave gates as you found them or as marked.

- Stay on the existing trail, and don't litter. Practice "Leave No Trace" on all trails.

- When hiking with children, use common sense to judge a child's capacity to hike a particular trail, and expect that the child may tire and need to be carried. Make sure children are adequately clothed for the weather, have proper shoes, and are protected from the sun with sunscreen and a hat. Kids dehydrate quickly, so make sure you have plenty of fluids for everyone.

- Take your time along the trails, whether you are doing one of this guide's short hikes or longer treks. In other words, don't miss the trees for the forest. You may finish some hikes long before or after the times suggested in the overview box.

- Participate in some online wildlife-observation counts. Cornell University's Lab of Ornithology operates **ebird.org,** where you can log in at no charge and submit bird lists or find out what's being seen at some of the areas' birding hot spots. A similar count is being done for butterflies at **wisconsinbutterflies.org/ butterflies/sightings.**

- Never spook animals, and give them plenty of space. An unannounced approach, a sudden movement, or a loud noise startles most animals, and a surprised animal can be dangerous.

- Be courteous to others you encounter on the trails.

- Look up! Keep an eye out for standing dead trees and storm-damaged living trees with loose or broken limbs that can fall at any time.

- Know your ability, and carry necessary supplies for changes in weather or other conditions.

TRAIL RECOMMENDATIONS

BEST HIKES FOR CHILDREN

BEST HIKES FOR BIRD-WATCHING

BEST HIKES ALONG WATERWAYS

WILDLIFE-VIEWING HIKES

DOG-FRIENDLY HIKES

WHEELCHAIR-ACCESSIBLE HIKES

BEST HIKES FOR WILDFLOWERS

BUSIEST HIKES ON WEEKENDS

BEST WINTER HIKES

All these hikes are great for the Houston area's temperate winter weather.

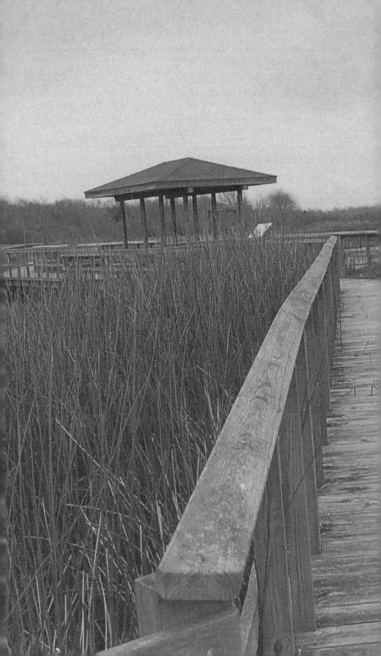

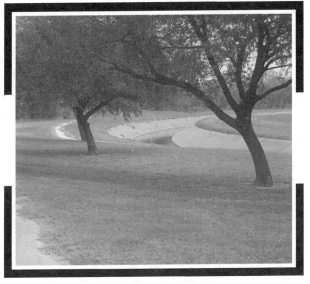

White Oak Bayou in Houston Heights

Urban Houston

Buffalo Bayou Park Hike and Bike Trail

■ OVERVIEW

LENGTH: 5.1 miles

CONFIGURATION: Loop

SCENERY: Woodlands, downtown Houston, bayou, cemetery, art sculptures, parkland

EXPOSURE: Sunny

TRAIL TRAFFIC: Light–moderate

TRAIL SURFACE: Asphalt and concrete

HIKING TIME: 2 hours

DRIVING DISTANCE: Inside the 610 Loop, about 4.8 miles from the intersection of Memorial Drive and the 610 Loop

ACCESS: Free

MAPS: USGS Houston Heights and Settegast

WHEELCHAIR ACCESS: Yes

FACILITIES: Parking, benches, water fountains, playground, canoe and kayak launches

SPECIAL COMMENTS: Close to downtown Houston, this hike covers an area that has been revitalized in the past few years. After heavy rains, be cautious of water levels in Buffalo Bayou, as it is one of the main flood-control channels in Houston and water levels stay high for days after a heavy rain.

MORE INFORMATION: (832) 395-7000, houstontx.gov/parks/trails.html

■ SNAPSHOT

This urban hike offers some great views of downtown Houston. As you hike west, away from the parking lot, you can see the new Federal Reserve Bank building to the south and new town homes on both sides of the bayou. Buffalo Bayou Park was originally created in 1929 to link downtown Houston with the suburban development of River Oaks, one of Houston's most affluent neighborhoods. The 124-acre park includes Eleanor Tinsley Park, the Police Officers Memorial, Glenwood Cemetery, Beth Yeshurun Cemetery, and the Sandy Reed Memorial Trail.

■ UP CLOSE

Once in the parking lot, head west toward Allen Parkway to get to the trail. Benches, a playground, and picnic tables are at Eleanor Tinsley Park, east of the parking lot. Head along the

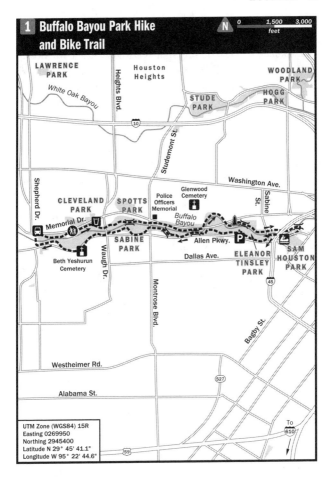

1 **Buffalo Bayou Park Hike and Bike Trail**

N

0   1,500   3,000
feet

LAWRENCE PARK

Houston Heights

WOODLAND PARK

White Oak Bayou

Heights Blvd.

STUDE PARK

HOGG PARK

10

Studemont St.

Washington Ave.

Shepherd Dr.

CLEVELAND PARK

SPOTTS PARK

Police Officers Memorial

Glenwood Cemetery

Sabine St.

Memorial Dr.

Buffalo Bayou

SABINE PARK

Allen Pkwy.

P

ELEANOR TINSLEY PARK

SAM HOUSTON PARK

Beth Yeshurun Cemetery

Waugh Dr.

Dallas Ave.

45

Montrose Blvd.

Bagby St.

Westheimer Rd.

527

Alabama St.

UTM Zone (WGS84) 15R
Easting 0269950
Northing 2945400
Latitude N 29° 45' 41.1"
Longitude W 95° 22' 44.6"

59

To 610

trail with Allen Parkway directly on your left and the park on your right. Most of the park is adorned with sculptures, making it one of the more eclectic urban parks in Houston. Cross the exit road from the parking lot and get back on the trail by going straight. Although the trail surface is concrete at the start, it changes to asphalt and stays this way for most of the hike. This is a hiking and biking trail, so be cautious of bikers. Stay to the right when hiking, and listen for bikers behind you.

Buffalo Bayou is on your right, between you and Memorial Drive to the north. Stay to the right on the trail, with Allen Parkway directly on your left. The trail heads right, away from the road, and down into the park. As it does, look to your left across Memorial Drive for the Police Officers Memorial, a monument dedicated to officers killed in the line of duty. Dedicated in 1992, the memorial is shaped like a cross and consists of five levels of stepped pyramids. To the west of the memorial is a granite stone etched with the names of the slain officers. Once into the park, the trail curves left beside benches and a planted garden. Past the garden, the trail swings right and takes you back to Allen Parkway. Hike along the road until it turns right and takes you closer to the bayou. Cross a bridge and head uphill. Although the bayou is on your right, its visibility is hampered greatly by overgrown kudzu vines, a plant that was brought from Japan in 1876 and heavily propagated throughout the South in the 1930s for foliage and to control soil erosion. It is one of the most invasive nonnative plants in the southeastern United States, growing up to a foot a day in the summer months and killing many native plants.

Buffalo Bayou Park is a popular dog and recreational park on weekends, but the trails remain only moderately used. Continue as the trail heads downhill and curves right among trees below the road. As the elevation changes, with the embankment on your left and the bayou on your right, the surroundings become much quieter. Cross another bridge and head uphill and left to a clearing on your left. Much of the park is mowed regularly, creating open green spaces, hills, and shade trees. As the trail winds back and forth, it heads uphill and then under Studemont Road. Past Studemont the trail swings left and uphill toward Allen Parkway. Large open spaces (and a few garbage cans) are on the right. The trail continues steeply uphill and then goes right, with a bench on the right and a railing on

the left between the trail and the road. Go past a water fountain on the left and a sign for the Waugh Drive Bat Colony.
About 250,000 Mexican free-tailed bats make the crevices of
the Waugh Drive bridge their permanent home—this is the
largest year-round bat colony in Texas. The bats can be seen
leaving the bridge to eat each evening just after dusk. After the
sign, head right and back into the park around a large geode-
sic water fountain. The trail passes the fountain and then heads
back uphill to Allen Parkway.

To the right is a metal fence separating the trail from the
bayou; before you reach Waugh Drive find a bat-viewing stand.
Take the right fork and follow the smell to go under Waugh
Drive; the presence of 250,000 bats makes for a very strong
odor. Go left after Waugh Drive and head back uphill toward
the road. After winding back and forth, the trail goes downhill
and curves right. Head back uphill and continue past the Beth
Yeshurun Cemetery, on your right. Follow the trail right and
back down into the park to a large green space, where you can-
not hear the road traffic. Continue past a bench on the left and
head back uphill by two benches on your right. At the intersection of Allen Parkway and Shepherd Drive, continue on
the trail, hiking along the Shepherd Drive bridge over Buffalo
Bayou. Once over the bridge, head right and past a Metro bus
stop to continue the hike. Memorial Drive is now on your left,
with the bayou on your right. Go past a water fountain on the
right and head downhill following the asphalt trail. The trail
surface, although narrower and older here, and perhaps covered in places with sand, is still easy to see.

Continue uphill toward Memorial Drive. A planted garden
to your right is followed by a sign for the Sandy Reed Memorial
Trail. Stop at the sign and look southwest to see the Beth Yeshurun
Cemetery across the bayou. Continue uphill, hiking by a bench
on the right and past another bat-colony sign. Go straight on the
trail past a set of stairs to the right. The trail swings right, taking
you beside the exit ramp for Waugh Drive. Take the right fork

to head back into the park, toward the bayou and under Waugh Drive. Discover another bat-viewing stand, and the undeniable smell of bats, before you reach the underpass. Hike under Waugh Drive and listen for high-pitched bat sounds. The trail curves right, past a water fountain on the left. High embankments on the left keep the traffic sounds away as you continue downhill.

Cross a bridge and hike past an exercise station on the right and a bench on the left. The trail starts back uphill past another bench and then under Studemont Road. The bayou is much more visible on your right as you go by a bench and head back downhill. As the trail bends left, go under Memorial Drive and hike about 150 yards before exiting and going left. The trail angles right; from here you can see the Police Officers Memorial over the trees to your right. Cross another bridge before heading back under Memorial Drive to get back to the park between Allen Parkway and Memorial Drive. The trail goes left and takes you under one of the sculptures that was created specifically for the park. Continue on the trail over two small bridges, and then go left past a disc-golf marker on the right. Stay on the trail past all exits to streets, parking lots, canoe and kayak launches, and other landmarks.

At the exit for Sabine Street, the trail surface changes to concrete and the landscape is better maintained. The section from Sabine Street to Bagby Street is part of a revitalization plan that was completed in late 2006 and includes new lights, trail surface, plantings, and artwork. Go under many of the downtown underpasses and past all intersections until you reach a bridge on the right that takes you back to the other side of the trail. Take a right once off the bridge and head west toward the parking lot. Go past a canoe and kayak launch on your right, and take the left fork up a set of stairs. Continue right after the stairs and then go straight toward the parking lot, which is only a few hundred yards ahead.

■ TO THE TRAILHEAD

From the intersection of the 610 Loop and Memorial Drive, go east on Memorial Drive 3 miles to Shepherd Drive, and turn right. At the first stoplight, turn left onto Allen Parkway. Go 2.4 miles to Bagby Street, passing the parking lot on the opposite side of Allen Parkway, and turn left. Turn left again at the first light to get back onto Allen Parkway, heading west. The parking lot is 0.5 miles ahead on the right. If you find the lot is full, park in one of the other lots along Allen Parkway or on a side street—do not park directly on Allen Parkway or Memorial Drive, as both are high-traffic roads.

■ MORE FUN

The downtown Houston entertainment district is within walking distance of the Sabine Street–Bagby Street section of the hike, along with the Aquarium, an amusement park, and restaurant. Minute Maid Park, home of the Houston Astros, and Toyota Center, home of the Houston Rockets and the Houston Aeros, are just east of the hike. Sam Houston and Tranquility parks are also east of Buffalo Bayou Park.

■ OVERVIEW

LENGTH: 2 miles	**WHEELCHAIR ACCESS:** Yes
CONFIGURATION: Loop	**FACILITIES:** Restrooms, baseball fields, picnic tables
SCENERY: Bayou, woodlands, downtown skyline	
	SPECIAL COMMENTS: This hike and bike trail starts in Stude Park next to the Stude Community Center. The park, which includes ball fields, a swimming pool, playground, and picnic tables, can be crowded during warm-weather months, but the trail is often less crowded than other parts of the park. Pets must be leashed at all times.
EXPOSURE: Sunny	
TRAIL TRAFFIC: Light	
TRAIL SURFACE: Asphalt and dirt	
HIKING TIME: 1 hour	
DRIVING DISTANCE: Inside the 610 Loop, 4.2 miles from the intersection of the 610 Loop West and I-10	
	MORE INFORMATION: (832) 395-7000, houstontx.gov/parks/trails.html
ACCESS: Free; open 6 a.m.–11 p.m.	
MAPS: USGS Houston Heights and Settegast	

■ SNAPSHOT

The White Oak Bayou watershed covers about 111 square miles and comprises three primary streams: White Oak Bayou, Little White Oak Bayou, and Cole Creek. The White Oak Bayou Hike and Bike Trail is in Houston Heights, one of the oldest neighborhoods in the city. Chosen for its higher elevation (23 feet higher than downtown Houston), Houston Heights was started in 1890 by Oscar Martin Carter, a self-made millionaire. He created a utopian neighborhood at a time when Houston was plagued with yellow fever and annual floods. Houston Heights was the location of residences, businesses, schools, open spaces for parks, libraries, civic clubs, and churches—all necessary elements for a close-knit community. Starting in the 1940s an exodus to the suburbs caused the neighborhood to deteriorate, and by 1970 the Heights was known for poverty and crime. In 1973

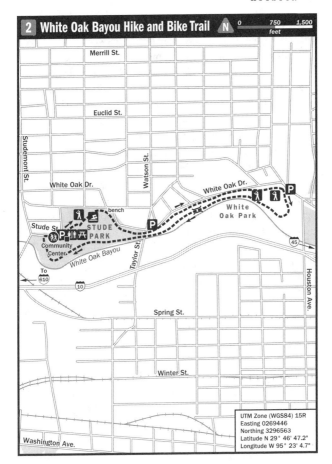

2 White Oak Bayou Hike and Bike Trail

Merrill St.

Euclid St.

Studemont St.

Watson St.

White Oak Dr.

White Oak Dr.

White
Oak Park

bench

Stude St.

STUDE
PARK

Community
Center.

White Oak Bayou

Taylor St.

To
610

10

Houston Ave.

45

Spring St.

Winter St.

Washington Ave.

UTM Zone (WGS84) 15R
Easting 0269446
Northing 3296563
Latitude N 29° 46' 47.2"
Longitude W 95° 23' 4.7"

the Houston Heights Association was established to revitalize
the community and preserve its historic buildings.

■ UP CLOSE

Start the hike from the parking lot across from the Stude
Community Center. Once on the asphalt trail, go left toward

the baseball fields and swimming pool. At the fork go right, past a bench on the left. You are now hiking between the baseball fields on your left and the swimming pool on the right. In the distance, to your right, is the downtown Houston skyline, just past I-10. Continue down the trail as it takes a right turn and then curves left. Go through the next intersection and then past another parking lot and bench on the left. More baseball fields come into view on the right as you hike gently downhill, past another bench on the left and toward some houses ahead.

As you get closer to White Oak Drive, the trail swings right. Continue past a bench and then the baseball fields, both on the right. Go past a bench on the left and then a third parking lot on the left, just across from the last baseball fields. As the trail heads away from the baseball fields, it goes downhill. At a fork bear left, keeping White Oak Bayou on your right. The sides of White Oak Bayou were hardened with concrete in the 1970s to control flooding—a common practice in Houston until the value of natural bayous was realized. As the trail heads uphill slightly, you pass under the Taylor Street underpass. Once past Taylor Street, the trail winds left and uphill, with houses on your left and the bayou still on your right. Although the right side of the trail has thick vegetation, this is a very sunny trail and you should wear sunscreen at all times.

Continue downhill and straight for some distance. As you pass an old park sign, look right to see a footbridge below in the flood overflow area of the bayou. You can also see a trail to your right—you'll use this to finish the hike. The area between the trail and bayou here is mowed, creating a large open area. Look far to your right for the freeway system that runs into Houston from the north. The trail continues to follow White Oak Drive and curves right. The area on the right contains thick vegetation, obscuring the view of the bayou. Head uphill steeply and continue through the next intersection. Look right for the overflow flood area of the bayou, which is overgrown with vegetation and also contains debris from recent floods. As you pass the King Biscuit Patio Cafe (a great local dining spot) on the left, head down the trail past a fence on the left. Take the right fork at the next intersection to head downhill and into the trees. The trail surface changes to dirt as you enter the bayou's overflow flood area. Go straight through the next intersection and then head right, following the trail. Downtown Houston is now on your left, and you are headed back in the direction you came from. Once you start back, the trail surface changes back to asphalt. At the intersection, take the right fork and go over a small spillway with a culvert for drainage.

White Oak Bayou is now on your left and a wooded area is on your right, just past a large swath of mowed grass. As the trail heads uphill, you can see the trail you came down earlier on the right. Go straight through the next intersection. The trail surface gets a little rough with eroded asphalt before changing back to smooth asphalt. As the trail narrows to no more than 3 feet wide, a high embankment on the left obscures views of downtown Houston. Continue as the trail bends right and downhill, allowing you to hike atop the concrete side of the bayou. Once off the concrete wall, the trail curves left and uphill. Cross a bridge over a small drainage channel, and then follow a winding course. Continue as the trail heads downhill and onto another part of the bayou's concrete wall before heading back under Taylor Street. Continue through the next intersection, past a bench on the right. The baseball fields are now on your right, with the bayou still on your left. The route heads uphill and through an intersection, with the community pool on your right. Go by two benches and then head steeply uphill toward a large sculpture. Stude Community Center and picnic tables are now on your right. The trail bends right, passing the sculpture and a playground, both right. Go past another bench on the right and continue toward the parking lot to finish the hike.

■ TO THE TRAILHEAD

From the 610 Loop West and I-10, drive 4 miles east to the Studemont exit. Turn left, go 0.25 miles to Stude Street, and turn right. The parking lot is straight ahead.

■ MORE FUN

Houston Arboretum & Nature Center and Memorial Park (page 32) are 3.5 miles west. The Galleria, one of the top shopping centers in the United States, is just west of the park, with downtown Houston to the east. Buffalo Bayou Park (page 12) and Tranquility Park are also close.

Terry Hershey Park: Cardinal, Mockingbird, and Blue Jay Trails

3

■ OVERVIEW

LENGTH: 4.8 miles

CONFIGURATION: Out-and-back and loop

SCENERY: Bayou, creek, open fields, woodlands, urban scenery

EXPOSURE: Sunny with some shade

TRAIL TRAFFIC: Light weekdays, moderate weekends

TRAIL SURFACE: Asphalt

HIKING TIME: 1.5 hours

DRIVING DISTANCE: 3.51 miles from the intersection of Beltway 8 and I-10

ACCESS: Free; open daily, 7 a.m.– 10 p.m.

MAPS: USGS Hedwig Village and Addicks; trail signs

WHEELCHAIR ACCESS: Yes

FACILITIES: Restrooms, parking, water fountains, dog fountains, benches, exercise stations, playground, runner's showers

SPECIAL COMMENTS: Pets, which must be leashed at all times, are welcome; dog water fountains are located wherever you see human water fountains. This trail is popular with cyclists and inline skaters; fortunately, it's wide enough to accommodate everyone.

MORE INFORMATION: (281) 496-2177, terryhersheypark.org

■ S N A P S H O T

Terry Hershey Park encompasses about 12.5 miles of trails, from TX 6 west to Beltway 8 east. The Cardinal, Mockingbird, and Blue Jay trails run from I-10 south and then west to TX 6. These three trails join to make one contiguous asphalt hiking and biking trail; however, no signs indicate when you have left one trail and started another, so make sure you look at the trail map at the parking lot to get your bearings. Restrooms are located on the Cardinal Trail shortly after starting the hike and again at the Eldridge Parkway end of the Blue Jay Trail.

■ U P   C L O S E

Once parked, go east toward a trail-map sign at the southeast corner of the parking lot. The trailhead for the Cardinal Trail starts just past the sign. The hike and bike trails are the main attractions in Terry Hershey Park, but other fun features include picnic sites, a playground, gazebos, a lighted walking trail along the Cardinal and Blue Jay trails, and a walk-in sundial near Memorial Drive and Eldridge Parkway. At the sundial, if you stand on the appropriate stone and the sun is shining, you cast a shadow on the correct time.

As you hike along South Mayde Creek and Buffalo Bayou, take note of the riparian landscape that includes plants such as yaupon holly, roughleaf dogwood, black willow, sunflowers, and sedges. In the spring look for passionflower, lantana, Turk's cap, and *Bidens*. This hike runs entirely along either South Mayde Creek or Buffalo Bayou and encompasses three different trails: Cardinal, Mockingbird, and Blue Jay.

Once on the trail, take the first fork right to get on the Cardinal Trail. Cross South Mayde Creek on a small bridge and take the next fork left, heading away from the freeway. Continue past a playground on the left and restrooms on your right. Behind the restrooms is a small pond with a fishing pier. Several benches, a gazebo, water fountains, a runner's shower, and a parking lot accommodate hikers, bikers, and picnickers. Take

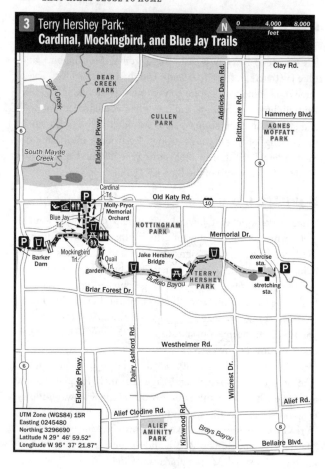

3 Terry Hershey Park:
Cardinal, Mockingbird, and Blue Jay Trails

the left fork in front of the parking lot and follow the trail along South Mayde Creek, on your left. This part of the hike, as well as the Blue Jay Trail, has lights for walking safely at dusk.

Continue along the trail to Memorial Drive. The creek can be quite deep here, with swift currents, so stay out of the water. Go under Memorial Drive and up the embankment to view one of the more urban parts of the trail. Once past Memorial Drive, the Cardinal Trail becomes the Blue Jay Trail. Just past several office buildings on the right, you eventually enter a more rural green space.

Stay away from the edge of the creeks and bayous, as the embankments are very steep and the sandy soil makes for unstable footing. The trails along the bayous often contain more elevation change than is typical in Houston, and the trails here are no exception. Continue past two benches and through a gated fence. The creek is left and houses are on your right. This part of the trail is exposed, so come prepared with sunscreen, hats, and plenty of water.

Soon the trees start to overarch the trail, creating needed shade. The most prevalent animals on this part of the hike are definitely squirrels—they are in the trees, on the ground, everywhere. Go past several benches and follow the trail left over a bridge. At the other end of the bridge is the trailhead for the Mockingbird Trail; turn right and begin the out-and-back part of the hike. Once on the Mockingbird Trail, Buffalo Bayou is on your right and open fields, or retention areas, are on your left.

Lights continue on this part of the trail but only for a short distance. At a fork, bear right, past a bench on the left. A high embankment on the left and the bayou on the right creates a tunnel, with trees as the roof. Continue over a bridge, walking beside an unofficial bike trail. Beyond a bench, the trail bends left. After a long straightaway, the trail swings right to cross a bridge. Cross two more bridges and go through a gate (closed and locked at night). The bayou is to the right, and if you look long enough, you may see an alligator swimming below.

Continue past a water fountain, under TX 6, and through parts of Barker Dam. Once up the other side of the dam, turn around and retrace 1.3 miles on the Mockingbird Trail. Where the Blue Jay and Mockingbird trails join, go straight. The Mockingbird and Blue Jay trails overlap for 0.3 miles.

While hiking, look for great blue herons, loggerhead turtles, and an occasional alligator. Other birds include ospreys, cardinals, herons, hawks, and killdeer along with wood ducks, warblers, cedar waxwings, and sparrows.

With Eldridge Parkway on your right, cross the bridge over Buffalo Bayou. (To find restrooms, follow the trail left and downhill, and then, at a fork, go left. Do not cross Eldridge Parkway.) To continue on the hike, take the right fork instead of the left. A trail map, along with a bench, is at this intersection. Go past a water fountain, bench, and runner's shower, noting the urban feel to this part of the hike. Town homes are to the right, with the bayou on the left. Ahead, a straight part of the trail has benches and picnic tables. Continue through this parklike area to an exercise station and nature sign on the right. The sign includes information on the trees found in the park, including cottonwood, green ash, pecan, live oak, sycamore, burr oak, and crepe myrtle. Just past the sign are a parking lot and benches on the right.

At a fork, bear left to cross under Memorial Drive, and transition from the Cardinal Trail to the Blue Jay Trail. Look as you cross under Memorial Drive for the trail you were on at the start of the hike. Continue past the Molly Pryor Memorial Orchard (dedicated to a Harris County clerk) on the left, a bench overlooking South Mayde Creek on the left, and two birdhouses on the right. Once past the last bench on the right, take the right fork back to the parking lot and the trailhead.

■ TO THE TRAILHEAD

From the intersection of Beltway 8 and I-10, head west 4.84 miles on I-10 to the TX 6 exit. Make a U-turn left by going under the freeway, and then go 1.33 miles on the access road to the entrance and parking lot of Terry Hershey Park, on the left.

4 Mercer Arboretum and Botanic Gardens: West Trails

■ OVERVIEW

LENGTH: 2.5 miles

CONFIGURATION: Loop

SCENERY: Woodlands, bald cypress stands, bog, creeks, wetlands, boardwalks, maple-tree collection

EXPOSURE: Shady with some sun

TRAIL TRAFFIC: Light

TRAIL SURFACE: Asphalt and boardwalk

HIKING TIME: 1 hour

DRIVING DISTANCE: 9.89 miles from the intersection of Beltway 8 and I-45

ACCESS: Free; in summer, M–Sa, 8 a.m.–7 p.m.; Su, 10 a.m.–7 p.m.; in winter, daily, 8 a.m.–5 p.m.

MAPS: USGS Spring; trail maps available on-site and at www.hcp4.net/mercer/pdf/mercermapInfo.pdf

WHEELCHAIR ACCESS: Yes

FACILITIES: Restrooms, arboretum, visitor center, parking, picnic areas, playgrounds, library, water fountains, trail markers

SPECIAL COMMENTS: Although most of the garden areas are accessible to wheelchairs and strollers, officials here ask that you call ahead for any special accommodations.

MORE INFORMATION: (281) 443-8731, www.hcp4.net/mercer

■ SNAPSHOT

Mercer, which is a nationally recognized arboretum and botanic garden, was preserved as a Harris County Precinct Park in 1974. Thelma and Charles Mercer presented the 250 acres along Cypress Creek to the county to create the region's largest collection of native and cultivated plants. This hike is on the west side of Aldine Westfield Road and includes many different trails and loops. The trails are well marked, and there are several restrooms. Look for deer and other wildlife, and be aware of poisonous snakes.

■ UP CLOSE

Start the hike at the trailhead adjacent to the dining pavilion, on the north side of the west parking lot. Restrooms are on the left, and the trail begins on a wooden boardwalk. Beyond the boardwalk, the trail surface changes to crushed granite and asphalt for the remainder of the hike. Before setting out, use bug spray for protection against both mosquitoes and horse-flies, which can bite through clothing. Continue onto the gran-ite walkway and past elderberry bushes on your left. Bear left at a fork, away from the parking lot and into the woods. A creek-bank erosion area is now on your right. Because of loose, sandy soil, you are advised to stay on the trail.

With the creek still on your right, bear right at a fork and continue through dense woodlands. At the next fork, bear right over a bridge. Continue through an intersection where a trail joins on the right. As you walk under a natural arbor, look left to see other trails. At an intersection, bear left to the Cypress Pond Loop and then take a right at a trailhead sign for that loop. A nature sign, left, describes quince trees. At a set of restrooms, take the left fork. Continue as the trail winds through Virginia mag-nolia, post oak, and hawthorn trees, which arch over the trail. Where the trail curves right, notice the bald cypresses growing in the creek on the right. Although they need a wet environment, they can survive droughts, which occur in the area regularly. Bald cypress is not a true cypress but more closely related to the coast redwood of California. These deciduous trees can grow to more than 90 feet tall and can live up to 1,000 years. They anchor themselves to wet creek beds with a root system that rises up and out of the water in the form of buttresses, or "cypress knees." Go past a bench on the right and head up the oxbow, an old channel of Cypress Creek that was left when the main channel moved far-ther north, perhaps during a flood. Streams and creeks relocate over long periods of time, changing their channels many times. These meanders are called oxbows and serve as overflow chan-nels for the creek during floods.

Continue along the trail and take the next fork right. Keep your eyes open for deer, which are frequently seen in this area. As the trail curves left, you pass a grassy clearing on

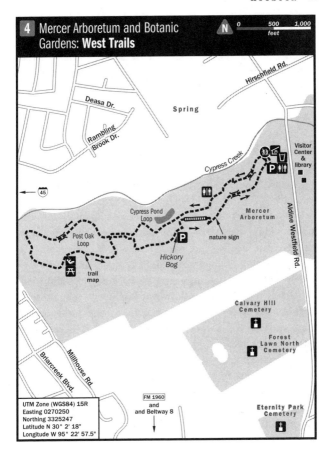

4 Mercer Arboretum and Botanic Gardens: **West Trails**

the right. The forest consists of tall trees and numerous vines that are killing many of them. Green moss grows on many of the lower parts of the trees, indicating a lack of sunlight and a persistently damp environment. At a fork marked by a sign for Hickory Bog, bear right. Continue past a bench and trail map on the right, and then take the next fork right to the Post Oak Loop. This loop includes gentle ridges that are well above the floodplain of Cypress Creek. These uplands are home to hardwood trees such as post oak and red oak. The trail is more shaded here, beneath a canopy of trees. Cross over a large bridge that curves right, and continue to the next trailhead and trail map. Continue straight to the Hawthorn Loop, where the trees get denser. Look for the cream-colored flowers of parsley hawthorn and pasture haw.

Continue straight through the next intersection. The Post Oak parking lot is now on your right, with another dining pavilion on the left. Take the next fork left at a trail sign, and continue past a playground, restrooms, and picnic areas. Go through the next intersection, where a trail joins on the right. At the end of the picnic area, continue straight past a trail map on the left and an intersection with a trail on the right. Immediately after leaving the picnic area, you are back in the woods. Swing left and slightly downhill to the next trailhead and map on the left. Go straight until you come to a sign for Hickory Bog, and then take the right fork. A mowed clearing is left, with the forest 30 yards or more away. Continue past more clearings until you get to a boardwalk and Hickory Bog, home to water hickory and water elm that have adapted to grow in seasonal wetlands. Also growing in the bog are water oak and Louisiana iris. Stay on the boardwalk, as snakes are more likely in wetlands. As you leave the boardwalk, the trail curves right. Go past a water fountain on the right and take the right fork at the next trailhead. Bald Cypress Swamp is straight ahead, with a long boardwalk, an observation stand, benches, and nature signs.

Follow the boardwalk to its end and exit left and back onto a crushed-granite surface. A parking lot is across the swamp, and a road is to your right. Take the next fork right and cross a bridge with benches at both ends. Ahead is the Jake Roberts Maple Collection, a stand of trident maples that produce a tunnel effect. In the fall, these maples change color, brilliantly creating beautiful autumn foliage in reds and oranges. Continue through the maple collection, past several benches, and take the next fork left. Pass a water fountain and several benches on your right, just this side of the parking lot. At the next intersection, fork right to get to the parking lot.

Note: All plants are protected and are not to be removed from the trails or gardens. The arboretum and botanic gardens are on both sides of Aldine Westfield Road, with the hiking trails located on the west side. The visitor center, botanic gardens, and library are all on the east side. Pets on leashes may visit the park on the west side only. Bikes are allowed on the asphalt trails of the west side. Swimming, ball playing, and other team sports are not permitted.

■ TO THE TRAILHEAD

From the intersection of Beltway 8 and I-45, head north 5.69 miles on I-45 to FM 1960 and turn right. Go 3 miles to Aldine Westfield Road and turn left. Go 1.2 miles to the entrance to Mercer Arboretum and Botanic Gardens. Turn left into the west side of the park to reach the trailhead. Take the first right and park in the Cypress parking lot on your immediate left, close to the dining pavilion on the north side of the lot.

5   Memorial Park: Cambodia Trail

■ OVERVIEW

LENGTH: 3.4 miles

CONFIGURATION: Out-and-back

SCENERY: Creek beds, woodlands, kudzu field

EXPOSURE: Shady

TRAIL TRAFFIC: Moderate

TRAIL SURFACE: Dirt

HIKING TIME: 2 hours

DRIVING DISTANCE: Inside the 610 Loop, 0.6 miles from the intersection of the 610 Loop and Woodway Drive

ACCESS: Free

MAPS: USGS Houston Heights; trail map available at trailhead

WHEELCHAIR ACCESS: No

FACILITIES: Restrooms, picnicking, baseball fields, trail signs

SPECIAL COMMENTS: The Cambodia Trail is heavily used on the weekends by cyclists but is used only sparingly during the week. This up-and-down trail can be challenging for someone with limited abilities but is still easily hiked by most people. The trail has numerous color-coded trail markers to help you navigate through the park. On weekends heavy car traffic is nearby, so any hiker with a respiratory condition should exercise caution.

MORE INFORMATION: (832) 395-7000, houstontx.gov/parks/memorialpark.html

■ SNAPSHOT

Memorial Park, the largest urban park in Texas, is often called the Central Park of Houston. It includes an 18-hole golf course, tennis courts, baseball and softball fields, football/soccer fields, picnic sites, a 3-mile jogging trail, a swimming pool, croquet, volleyball, inline skating, cycling, and hiking. The 1,600-acre park was acquired by William C. Hogg from the U.S. government in 1918; he subsequently turned it over to the City of Houston. The park already contains many hiking and biking trails, with more being added over a five-year period that began in 2008. All the wooded areas on the south side of the park are crisscrossed by trails, many of which run along Buffalo Bayou and other, smaller creeks. The Cambodia Trail starts from the

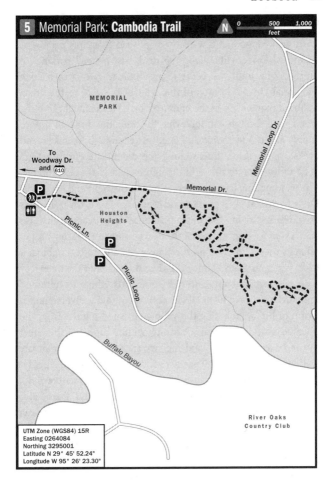

5 Memorial Park: **Cambodia Trail**

N   0   500   1,000
                feet

MEMORIAL
PARK

To
Woodway Dr.
and 610

Memorial Dr.

Memorial Loop Dr.

Houston
Heights

Picnic Ln.

Picnic Loop

Buffalo Bayou

River Oaks
Country Club

UTM Zone (WGS84) 15R
Easting 0264084
Northing 3295001
Latitude N 29° 45' 52.24"
Longitude W 95° 26' 23.30"

next entrance off Memorial Drive, but because this entrance is
often closed, park at the entrance directly past the second stoplight and walk east toward the start of the trail. Restrooms and
water fountains are near the parking lots.

■ UP CLOSE

Once parked, go east toward the park road that runs parallel to Memorial Drive. Hike along the road, past a small parking lot on the right, until you come to an entrance gate farther along Memorial Drive. Go around the front of the gate to the green trailhead marker across the entrance road. Head straight into the woods and then go left, following the trail. The dirt trail surface is only about 3 feet wide and is not wide enough for hikers and cyclists at the same time, so look ahead and listen from behind at all times. Step to the right if you see or hear a cyclist coming. The winding trail has a deep creek bed to the right and Memorial Drive to the left. As it goes toward Memorial Drive, the trail heads downhill and right. This descent is quite steep in some areas, so watch your footing and take it slowly if you are not wearing proper hiking shoes. Continue on the trail uphill and to the right as it takes you away from Memorial Drive and back into the trees.

These mixed pine-and-oak woodlands, which are hemmed in by urban sprawl from all directions, contain a diverse population of birds, including the yellow-crowned night heron, the pileated woodpecker, and, during winter months, the great horned owl. Pine, oak, and hickory trees border most of the trail; you can also find parsley hawthorn, American beautyberry, snowdrop tree, sweet bay magnolia, eastern redbud, Texas mountain laurel, coral honeysuckle, coral bean, and southern wax myrtle. Animals to watch for include Virginia opossums, gray squirrels, eastern moles, fox squirrels, evening bats, nine-banded armadillos, raccoons, swamp rabbits, and coyotes; coral snakes and copperheads are also found here, so give them a wide berth if you encounter them.

Go past a trail marker on your left and one on your right. Follow the marker on your right to head back into the trees, with the creek bed on your right. The ground on the left goes uphill, away from the trail. The trail narrows slightly, so be extra-vigilant about watching for cyclists. Continue past another trail marker and go left and downhill over numerous tree roots. As the trail takes a big bend to the right, go through the next intersection heading straight ahead. At the next trail marker on the left, continue straight. The trail winds right and then sharply left, with a lot of accumulated sand on the trail surface. Head downhill and then back up the other side of the hill, hiking over tree roots and packed dirt. At the next intersection, go left. Cyclists like to take the steeper right fork, but it's best for hikers to take the high embankment on the left. Continue straight at the next intersection where the two trails meet.

The trail bends sharply left and uphill over an eroded stretch. The center of the trail is at least 2 feet below the sides. The trail then curves right, with the creek bed still on your right. You can still clearly hear the traffic on Memorial Drive, to your left. Continue past a trail marker on your right and go straight to stay on the trail. Numerous vines hang from the trees, and the vegetation is thick; however, visibility into the trees is good. Go past another trail marker on the left and head downhill over another eroded part of the trail. Once downhill, go to the right and head back uphill. The trail continues to wind back and forth, going uphill and downhill many times before coming to another trail marker on the right. Head downhill and to the right, past the marker. Go uphill and follow the trail as it winds over big tree roots. Pass another trail marker on the right. The trail, which levels somewhat, is not quite so up-and-down here. Go between two trees—hard for a bike but quite easy on foot. As the trail takes a big turn to the left, it heads downhill before leveling again.

Continue past another marker as you step up and over a small embankment. The trail takes a quick left and then goes right, heading downhill. A big bend left takes the trail uphill. Head slightly left to stay on the trail, and then climb steeply upward. Go around a fallen tree and then head right. Cross a small bridge and keep following the trail as it winds back and forth. After another big bend to the left, the trail heads uphill gradually to another trail marker on the right. Go straight to the next trail marker and a sign on the right that states NO BIKES BEYOND THIS POINT. After the sign, the trail winds left and then right, passing more NO BIKES signs on the left. The trail is much flatter here, with little elevation change. Continue straight past another trail marker on the right. As the trail curves left, it narrows some. Hike past a nursery on your left and follow the marker on the right. The trail takes a big right turn before going past two benches and another trail marker. Go right onto a narrower part of the trail and then past another trail marker on the right before a big bend to the left.

Walk over a fallen tree in the middle of the trail, past a marker on the right and another NO BIKES sign. Continue past another marker and NO BIKES sign as the trail winds back and forth, downhill and then back uphill. As the trail bends right and then takes a quick left, head downhill steeply. Look to your right and you can see the trail that you will be on shortly. Hike past more NO BIKES signs on the left and some houses that you can see just over the trees on the left. As the trail swings back to the right, head away from the creek bed and into an opening with a trail marker pointing straight ahead. Go straight into a large field of overgrown kudzu, a plant that was brought over from Japan in 1876 and heavily propagated throughout the South in the 1930s to control soil erosion. It is one of the most invasive nonnative plants in the southeastern United States, growing up to a foot a day in summer and killing many native plants. Head through the kudzu on both sides of the trail to the next intersection, and take the left fork. Head downhill steeply and to the right before going back to the left. Go straight up the trail over rocks and dirt as you leave the kudzu field. At the next intersection, keep left until you come to the opening you were in at the start of the kudzu field. Head to the right at the inter-section and hike back up the trail the same way you came.

■ TO THE TRAILHEAD

From the 610 Loop and Woodway Drive, drive 0.6 miles west to the second stoplight. Turn right and then left. Parking is available on both sides of the Memorial Park Picnic Loop.

■ MORE FUN

Houston Arboretum & Nature Center, (713) 681-8433, is only 0.25 miles west of the trailhead, off Woodway Drive. Additional Memorial Park amenities include a golf course, (713) 862-4033; tennis center, (713) 867-0440; and swimming and fitness center, (713) 802-1662. The Galleria, one of the top shopping centers in the United States, is just west of the park, with downtown Houston to the east. Buffalo Bayou Park (page 12), White Oak Bayou Hike and Bike Trail (page 18), and Tranquility Park are also close by.

6   Jesse H. Jones Park: East Trails

■ OVERVIEW

LENGTH: 2.2 miles

CONFIGURATION: Loop with short out-and-back

SCENERY: Woodlands, drainage channel, wetlands, Akokisa Indian Village

EXPOSURE: Shady

TRAIL TRAFFIC: Light weekdays, moderate weekends

TRAIL SURFACE: Asphalt

HIKING TIME: 1 hour

DRIVING DISTANCE: 12.36 miles from the intersection of Beltway 8 and US 59

ACCESS: Free; open Mar–Oct, 8 a.m.–7 p.m.; Nov and Feb, 8 a.m.–6 p.m.; Dec and Jan, 8 a.m.–5 p.m.

MAPS: USGS Maedan; trail maps available on-site and at www.hcp4.net/jones/pdf/trailmap.pdf

WHEELCHAIR ACCESS: Yes

FACILITIES: Restrooms, nature center, parking, picnic areas, playgrounds, fishing on Spring Creek, historical sites

SPECIAL COMMENTS: Children under age 12 must be supervised at all times, and no pets are allowed in the park. Venomous snakes, fire ants, and poison ivy are found along the trails, so stay alert and on-trail. Park rules prohibit hiking off the developed trails. Fishing is allowed in Spring Creek only.

MORE INFORMATION: (281) 446-8588, www.hcp4.net/jones

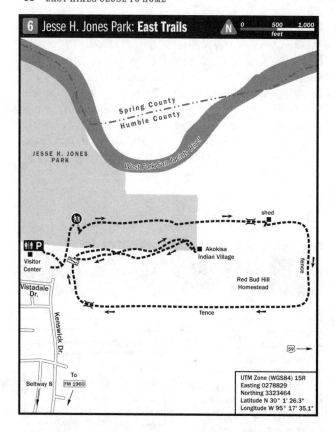

6 Jesse H. Jones Park: **East Trails**

0   500   1,000
feet

Spring County
Humble County

JESSE H. JONES
PARK

West Fork San Jacinto River

shed

Akokisa
Indian Village

Red Bud Hill
Homestead

fence

fence

Visitor
Center

Vistadale
Dr.

Kensick Dr.

59

To
Beltway 8   FM 1960

UTM Zone (WGS84) 15R
Easting 0278829
Northing 3323464
Latitude N 30° 1' 26.3"
Longitude W 95° 17' 35.1"

■ SNAPSHOT

The East Trails hike at Jesse H. Jones Park uses the Jones Bender and Homestead trails. The Jones Bender Trail starts and ends at the first parking lot on the right. The Homestead Trail, in the middle of the Jones Bender Trail, is an out-and-back that leads to Redbud Hill Homestead and Akokisa Indian Village. Redbud Hill is a re-creation of an 1820–1830 East Texas homestead with a log cabin, smokehouse, root cellar, chicken house, garden, bread oven, privy, woodworking shop, blacksmith shop, barn, and corral. Akokisa

Indian Village, adjacent to the homestead, comprises a hut, chickee, lean-to, sweat lodge, and council lodge. Both are open for self-guided tours on Wednesdays and Saturdays, 1–4 p.m.

■ UP CLOSE

The East Trails hike starts from the first parking lot on your right as you enter the park. Hike toward the Homestead Trail sign and head left to the trailhead for the Jones Bender Trail. This trail is part of the Spring Creek Greenway project, which has created trails throughout Jesse H. Jones Park, and is the only trail in the park open to bikes on weekdays only. The asphalt surface runs along a riparian floodplain ecosystem. Continue on the trail to the first nature sign, pointing out the Texas sugarberry tree, noted for the corky warts found on its bark. Go through an intersection where a trail joins on the left.

Nature signs supply information on the plants in the area. One of the first signs is for water oak, the most common oak in the floodplain forest. Water oaks and pines form a canopy over the 10-foot-wide trail. The trail can accommodate hikers and cyclists at the same time; just remember to hike on the right to give bikes room to pass. Another nature sign points out sweet gum, which can reach heights of up to 80–150 feet. These trees are characterized by the spiny, gumball-like structures that hang until ripe and then fall to the ground. Other trees in the park include cedar elm, water hickory, yaupon and American holly, and red oak.

Continue past a small creek on the left and up a steep incline as the trail heads toward a flood-control channel. Go through an intersection with a trail on the right and a bench on the left. Look for opossums, raccoons, armadillos, swamp rabbits, coyotes, bobcats, deer, and beavers at the flood-control channel, built for area neighborhoods. Birds include the pileated and red-bellied woodpeckers, red-shouldered hawk, barred owl, mockingbird, and wood duck. More than 30 kinds of snakes call the park home, but only the copperhead, coral, and cottonmouth are poisonous.

The bridge over the drainage channel is the only open part of the hike; otherwise, the trail is almost exclusively under the canopy of trees. Once across the bridge, a nature-viewing blind on the left has small slits in the wall facing the water and the wetlands below. Continue hiking uphill, where the forest floor gets denser on both sides of the trail. The trail nears the park-boundary fence on your left with dense forest on your right. As the trail starts downhill, the forest floor on the right opens considerably with young trees. Soon the trail curves right, taking you back west. The fence, which continues to be on the left, is now the boundary for the south side of the park. The forest floor gets denser as the trail continues to head downhill.

Continue down the hill past a bench and into another section of the flood-control channel, where a large birdhouse and wetlands appear on the right. The drainage channel, although artificial, has created a wetland habitat for egrets, herons, ibises, plovers, and sandpipers. Several species of dragonflies may also be found hovering nearby. Hike up the other side of the drainage channel and back onto the shaded trail, past very dense undergrowth on the right. A nature sign for post oak, a member of the white-oak family, is on the right. Now go through an intersection where a trail joins on the right. The vegetation on the left is very thick, but the right side has opened, allowing better visibility into the woods. Cross a small bridge and continue down the trail.

The trail curves past a neighborhood swimming pool and tennis courts, both left. The park-boundary fence is still on the left but now marks the west side of the park. Continue as the trail descends and curves left, allowing you to see the parking lot up ahead. Exit the Jones Bender Trail and bear right through the parking lot to the trailhead for the Homestead Trail. Take a right out of the parking lot to get on the 0.6-mile out-and-back trail and go through a wooden gate. The trail surface is now crushed granite and continues to be very wide. A bench is on the right where the trail swings right. The forest floor is very open, as the understory vegetation does not get enough sunlight to allow for much growth. Continue past a nature sign for greenbrier, a root food source for Native Americans. Considerable moss is on the trees, indicating that the area stays moist.

Bear left at an intersection and then go straight through the next one. Park-maintenance buildings are about 75 yards to the right. Continue past a nature sign describing Hercules club, known as the toothache tree because of its numbing effects when applied to an afflicted area. Go past a bench on the right and an old wood fence on the left. The trail curves right and into the Redbud Hill Homestead and Akokisa Indian Village. Early-18th-century explorers encountered the Akokisa, who lived in a large village just across Spring Creek from the present-day park. By the 1850s the Akokisa had either merged with other tribes in the area or had died from European diseases. The village re-creation shows that they were skilled at making dugout canoes from cypress logs and tanning bear hides.

At the homestead and village, turn around and retrace the Homestead Trail. At a fork, bear left; a nearby nature sign describes Alabama supplejack and sassafras. Take the next left fork, past a bench on your right. The hike soon ends at the Homestead Trail trailhead and the parking lot.

Note: Bicycles are allowed on most hiking trails only on Sundays, 8 a.m.–noon, except on the Jones Bender Trail, where they are also permitted during the week (but not on Saturday).

■ TO THE TRAILHEAD

From the intersection of Beltway 8 and US 59, head north 4.66 miles on US 59 to FM 1960 and turn left. Go 1.7 miles to Kenswick Drive and turn right. Go 1 mile to the end of the road and the entrance to the park. Park headquarters are immediately on your left as you enter. The parking lot is on your right.

■ MORE FUN

The park offers guided nature and pioneer tours for school groups. The nature center is open year-round, 8 a.m.–4:30 p.m., except when the park is closed. Call ahead to ensure that it is open. Lake Houston Park is just a few miles north, off US 59.

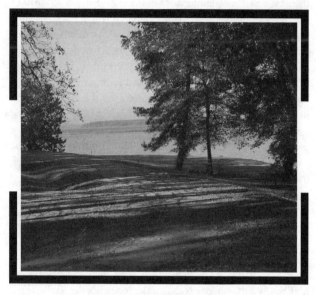

A view of Lake Livingston from the trail

State Parks near Houston

■ O V E R V I E W

LENGTH: 4.2 miles

CONFIGURATION: Out-and-back

SCENERY: Big Thicket, woodlands, cypress swamps, creeks, sloughs

EXPOSURE: Shady

TRAIL TRAFFIC: Light

TRAIL SURFACE: Dirt and sand

HIKING TIME: 2 hours

DRIVING DISTANCE: 82 miles from the junction of Beltway 8 and I-10

ACCESS: $2 per person age 13 and older; open 8 a.m.–10 p.m.

MAPS: USGS Silsbee; trail maps available at park headquarters and at the Web site below (click "Map of Park" at left)

WHEELCHAIR ACCESS: No

FACILITIES: Restrooms, parking, campsites, picnic tables, playground, water fountains, showers, cabins, canoe rental and shuttle service by local outfitters

SPECIAL COMMENTS: Pets must be on a leash (6 feet or shorter) at all times.

MORE INFORMATION: (409) 755-7322, tpwd.state.tx.us/spdest/findadest/parks/village_creek

■ S N A P S H O T

The Water Oak Trail takes you through the southern part of Village Creek State Park. This wide, relatively flat, and easily hiked trail has changed dramatically since Hurricane Rita. The vegetation is much sparser, creating a sunnier hike with much more forest-floor plants than before. The park, which opened in 1994, contains 1,090 acres and borders Village Creek. Various tours and interpretative programs are available throughout the year and can be found on the Texas Parks and Wildlife events calendar (**tpwd.state.tx.us/newsmedia/calendar**). The town of Lumberton, only minutes away, can furnish groceries and fishing supplies.

■ U P   C L O S E

To start the hike, park in the lot just past the bridge. Come out of the parking lot on the park road to the left, continuing past the bike trail sign on the left. Pass an open area on your right

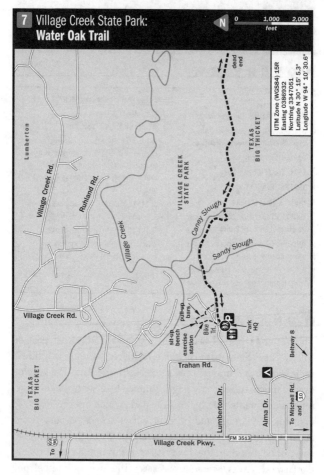

7 Village Creek State Park: Water Oak Trail

N

0   1,000   2,000
feet

UTM Zone (WGS84) 15R
Easting 0386932
Northing 3347051
Latitude N 30° 15' 5.3"
Longitude W 94 ° 10' 30.6"

dead end

Lumberton

Village Creek Rd.

Ruhland Rd.

Village Creek

VILLAGE CREEK
STATE PARK

TEXAS
BIG THICKET

Caney Slough

Sandy Slough

Village Creek Rd.

pull-up bars

sit-up
bench
exercise
station

Bike Trl.

Park HQ

Beltway 8

TEXAS
BIG THICKET

Trahan Rd.

Lumberton Dr.

Alma Dr.

To Mitchell Rd.
and (10)

To (69)(96)

Village Creek Pkwy.

FM 3513

where many of the native trees were destroyed by Hurricane Rita in 2005. Before the storm there were no open areas in this park, and visibility into the forest was scarce due to the thick vegetation. At the first intersection, turn right, following signs for the Water Oak Trail. Go past motorized-vehicle barriers and continue down the sandy trail. It's about 12 feet wide and can be a bit difficult to hike due to deep sand. The vegetation on the left is thick, and a small creek runs on the right. Pass a maintenance yard on the right, and continue straight. Because the trail is sandy, you may be able to identify animal tracks, such as those made by deer, bobcats, and raccoons.

As you hike, notice the cypress, water tupelo, river birch, mayhaw, water oak, loblolly pine, and yaupon trees. Because the park is part of the floodplain of the Neches River, baygalls and backwater sloughs are also running throughout the area. Baygalls are areas that developed along sandy-bottom small streams. The term often refers to the stream itself and the vegetation along it, or both. Wildlife is abundant and includes snapping turtles, diamondback water snakes, coral snakes, speckled king snakes, bobcats, raccoons, white-tailed deer, opossum, armadillos, coyotes, and wild hogs. More than 200 species of birds are native to the Texas Big Thicket; expect to find wood ducks, egrets, herons, pileated woodpeckers, yellow-billed cuckoos, roadrunners, and painted buntings, just to name a few. Fishing in Village Creek State Park is permitted, so you can try your luck for catfish, bass, perch, and panfish.

Continue straight through an intersection with the Bike Trail. The Water Oak Trail heads slightly uphill and winds left. Then it narrows and the sand surface changes to packed dirt, making for an easier hike. The vegetation is thick on both sides of the trail, but evidence of past hurricanes is still noticeable. Go through the next intersection, where a trail joins on the left. Cross Sandy Slough, a small waterway that may be dry depending on the time of year. If water is in the slough, you can rock-hop across. The trail heads uphill and right before taking a big leftward bend. At the bend, you'll notice that many of the trees in this area are gone. Go past a trailhead on the left and continue straight. Soon the trail narrows to about 6 feet wide and loses its roadlike appearance. At the next intersection, angle right. The trail heads uphill and left, winding past yaupon and water oak as it becomes much shadier. Soon you'll find a cypress swamp with exposed "knees" on your right and Caney Slough on your left. Cross a small creek bed and go past a sign on the right pointing out the champion Texas river birch. Go past a yellow marker in a tree on the left and continue along a curvy course. The trail surface changes from dirt to sand, indicating the presence of the slough that runs along the left side of the trail. As the water in the slough rises, the sand migrates over to the trail surface.

At the Caney Slough sign, cross a bridge and then go straight to get back on the trail. Look left for a beaver swamp. The trail curves left and then takes a big rightward bend as you head to an intersection with the Yaupon Loop Trail. Continue straight through the intersection to where the trail dead-ends at the park boundary. Turn around and retrace your route to the parking lot.

■ TO THE TRAILHEAD

From the intersection of Beltway 8 and I-10 East, head east 69 miles on I-10 to the TX 69/96 North exit in Beaumont. Go 12 miles on TX 69/96 to the Mitchell Road exit. Exit and go 0.4 miles on the access road; then turn right on Mitchell Road. Turn immediately left onto FM 3513 and go 2 miles to Alma Drive. Turn right, cross the railroad tracks, and go 0.5 miles to the park entrance, on the left. Park directly next to the park headquarters.

■ MORE FUN

The Big Thicket National Preserve Visitor Center, (409) 951-6700, is 20 miles north on Highway 96. Also in the area are Sea Rim State Park (tpwd.state.tx.us/spdest/findadest/parks/sea_rim); Cattail Marsh, in Beaumont's Tyrrell Park, (409) 861-1929; and Pleasure Island (pleasureislandtx.com), an artificial island near Port Arthur with fishing, golf, biking, and more. Museums in Beaumont include the Fire Museum of Texas (firemuseumoftexas.org), John Jay French House (jjfrench.com), McFaddin-Ward House (mcfaddin-ward .org), Texas Energy Museum (texasenergymuseum.org), and Clifton Steamboat Museum (cliftonsteamboatmuseum.com).

8 Stephen F. Austin State Park: Main Loop

■ OVERVIEW

LENGTH: 3 miles	**MAPS:** USGS San Felipe; trail maps available at park headquarters and at the Web site below (click "Trails Map" at left)
CONFIGURATION: Loop	
SCENERY: Forest, campgrounds, creek beds, golf course	
EXPOSURE: Partly shaded–very shaded	**WHEELCHAIR ACCESS:** No
TRAIL TRAFFIC: Light weekdays, moderate weekends	**FACILITIES:** Restrooms, picnic tables, campsites, showers, state-park store, trail signs
TRAIL SURFACE: Dirt and some overgrown grassy areas	**SPECIAL COMMENTS:** Dogs must be leashed at all times. Please be aware of poisonous snakes and a large population of deer.
HIKING TIME: 1.5 hours	
DRIVING DISTANCE: 36 miles from the intersection of Beltway 8 and I-10	
ACCESS: Day use, $3 per person age 13 and older, or buy a yearly Texas State Parks Pass; open 8 a.m.–10 p.m.	**MORE INFORMATION:** (979) 885-3613, tpwd.state.tx.us/ spdest/findadest/parks/ stephen_f_austin_and_san_felipe

■ SNAPSHOT

Stephen F. Austin State Park is bordered on the north and east by the Brazos River, which provides a habitat for many native plants and animals. While most of the park has been developed for camping, the undeveloped areas are great for hiking and fishing. During the week there is very little activity in the park, allowing for undisturbed hiking. Just east of the park is an 18-hole golf course that is part of the state-park system and operated by the Stephen F. Austin Golf Association.

■ UP CLOSE

Turn right out of the parking lot, walk up the road for about 100 feet, and locate the trailhead to your left. Cross the road to find the trailhead. At the trailhead, you can see the Stephen F. Austin Golf Course on your right and the park road on your

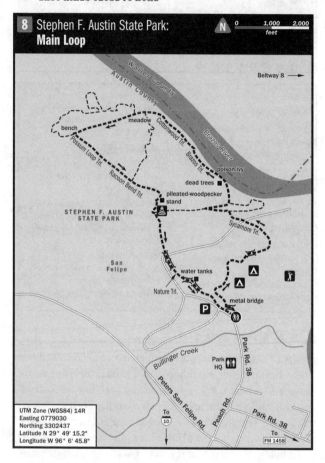

8 Stephen F. Austin State Park:
Main Loop

N

0   1,000   2,000
feet

Waller County
Austin County
Brazos River
Beltway 8 →

meadow
Cottonwood Trl.
bench
Brazos Trl.
Possum Loop Trl.
poison ivy
Racoon Bend Trl.
dead trees
pileated-woodpecker
stand

STEPHEN F. AUSTIN
STATE PARK

Sycamore Trl.

San
Felipe

water tanks

Nature Trl.

metal bridge

P

Bullinger Creek

Park
HQ

Park Rd. 38

Peters San Felipe Rd.

Peach Rd.

Park Rd. 38

To
10

To
FM 1458

UTM Zone (WGS84) 14R
Easting 0779030
Northing 3302437
Latitude N 29° 49' 15.2"
Longitude W 96° 6' 45.8"

left. About 20 feet along the trail is a fork. Bear right here, down
into a creek ravine.

At the bottom of the ravine, cross a metal bridge and start
back up the other side of the creek. Be aware that if it is rain-
ing, even a small creek can turn into a flash flood fairly quickly.
Once out of the ravine, the trail becomes quite primitive and
less well defined. The trail continues in and out of several creek

beds and through grassy, overgrown areas. The trail is very narrow and winding but still easy to follow. Watch out for large
spiderwebs from spring through early fall. Some of the spiders are banana spiders (also called yellow golden spiders),
which can grow up to 4 inches in diameter and can seem quite
menacing; they are not poisonous, however. The webs are gen-
erally about head-high, so you can duck below most of them.

Although the trail is still quite primitive, you can navigate
by watching for the large concrete blocks that have been placed
on it to help hikers maneuver through low-lying areas. Beyond
the first set of blocks, the trail is grassy and weedy, and the canopy opens to allow sunlight. The trail becomes more defined as
you cross a small bridge. The golf course is still visible on the
right, and campsites are visible on the left. The main loop trail
continues to alternate between primitive and defined. Be careful of the poison ivy, oak, and sumac that grow prodigiously
in this part of Texas. As you continue along the trail, the golf
course fades out of sight while the campsites continue to be
visible on your left. Cross another small stream, walking on
concrete "stones" in the creek bed, and hike back up the other
side. Once you're away from the creek, a water-treatment plant
becomes visible on your right. After you cross another creek
and hike through long grass, the trail opens. When you reach
a fork, bear left to access the trailhead for the Sycamore Trail.
You are now about a mile into the hike, on a dirt surface that
becomes wider and more maintained the farther along you go.

Once on the Sycamore Trail, head downhill for about 40
yards to a ravine, then climb uphill. This part of the trail is shady
and well maintained. At the next fork, bear left. The trail now
is reminiscent of a path through an antebellum estate: straight,
wide, shaded, and very pleasant. Even in August, this area is
considerably cooler than other parts of the park. Soon the trail
becomes more winding and the flora become more lush.

Now deep into the woods and in the undeveloped part of
the park, go left at the next fork, where the trail surface changes

to leaf-flecked dirt. Cross over several dead trees that have fallen over the trail. Poison ivy vines may be present here; to identify them, remember the Scout motto: "If it's hairy, it's scary." The fuzzy vines, like the leaves, cause a rash if touched, so take care to avoid them as you step under or over the fallen trees.

At the intersection, turn right onto the Brazos Bend Trail. Even wider and more pleasing than the Sycamore Trail, this trail is often used by Scout groups, so it could get a bit crowded on weekends during autumn and spring. Once on the Brazos Bend Trail, you leave the creek beds for good and head uphill to a flat part of the trail. At an intersection, continue straight to stay on the Brazos Bend Trail. Look high for scissor-tailed fly-catchers and pileated woodpeckers, and low for deer, raccoons, foxes, opossums, and squirrels.

Where the Brazos Bend Trail ends, take a left onto the Cottonwood Trail. Surrounded by large oaks and pecan trees, listen for the very loud, quick, staccato drumming of the pileated woodpecker high above. This straight trail heads uphill to a bench and the next intersection, where you turn left. This is the only steep hill in the park; if the trail is muddy and slippery, use the wooden steps to the left. Past the bench, the trail becomes roadlike, with even a trace of asphalt on some sections. Continue past the Possum Loop and Raccoon Bend trails, both left. At a fork, bear right. A pileated-woodpecker stand is set up for viewing, with benches and a viewing wall containing cut-outs at varying levels. Just past the stand is a small amphitheater, on the right. The trail goes left of the amphitheater and joins the park road. Turn right on the road and go past campsites, left, to where a road joins on the left. Cross the park road on your left and regain the trail.

This part of the trail is well maintained, taking you over several newly constructed wooden bridges. Go through the Nature Trail intersection and continue down the trail. Cross one last bridge and bear right at the next fork to the parking lot and the end of the hike.

Note: The first mile of the trail is very primitive, so wear long pants. Along this stretch, look for spiders and webs anywhere two trees flank the path. For a more groomed trail, start this hike at the Sycamore trailhead.

■ TO THE TRAILHEAD

From Beltway 8 and I-10, head west on I-10 for 33 miles. Exit and turn right onto FM 1458. Drive 2 miles to Park Road 38 and turn left. The park entrance is 1 mile ahead, at the end of the road. From the park headquarters, take Park Road 38 straight and park in the first lot on the left.

■ MORE FUN

San Felipe de Austin State Historic Site, operated by the Texas Historical Commission, is across FM 1458 from the state park. San Felipe is where Stephen F. Austin brought the first 297 families to colonize Texas in 1824. It was the capital of the American colonies in Texas and is called the "Cradle of Texas Liberty," as the conventions of 1832 and 1833 and the Consultation of 1835 were held here. These meetings led to the Texas Declaration of Independence. San Felipe is home to the first settler newspaper (the *Texas Gazette*), the home of the Texas postal system, and the original home of the Texas Rangers. Historical tours are given every Saturday and Sunday at 1 p.m. For more information, call (979) 798-2202 or go to **visitsanfelipedeaustin.com.** At the entrance to the park is the 18-hole Stephen F. Austin Golf Course.

■ OVERVIEW

LENGTH: 3.8 miles

CONFIGURATION: 2 loops

SCENERY: Wetlands, lakes, Big Creek, woodlands, prairie

EXPOSURE: Sunny

TRAIL TRAFFIC: Light weekdays, moderate weekends

TRAIL SURFACE: Dirt and grass

HIKING TIME: 2 hours

DRIVING DISTANCE: 25.14 miles from the intersection of Beltway 8 and US 59

ACCESS: $4 per person, age 13 and older; open 8 a.m.–10 p.m. in summer and 8 a.m.–5 p.m. in winter

MAPS: USGS Thompsons and Otey; trail signs; trail maps available at park headquarters and at the Web site below (click "Map of Trails" at left)

WHEELCHAIR ACCESS: No

FACILITIES: Restrooms, parking, water fountains, dog fountains, benches, camping, picnic areas, playgrounds, fishing piers

SPECIAL COMMENTS: Pets welcome as long as they're leashed. The trail is wide enough to accommodate both hikers and bikers comfortably.

MORE INFORMATION: (979) 553-5102, tpwd.state.tx.us/spdest/findadest/parks/brazos_bend

■ SNAPSHOT

Brazos Bend State Park has more than 22 miles of hiking trails within its roughly 5,000 acres. Less than an hour from Houston, it is one of the best camping and day-use parks in the area. The Big Creek Loop Trail departs from the Horseshoe Lake Loop Trail and extends to the park boundary. More than 290 species of birds have been sighted here. A nature center, near the center of the park, houses exhibits that pertain to the major ecosystems (marshes and woodlands) in the vicinity. The center is open on weekends and most holidays 9 a.m.–5 p.m.; admission is free of charge. Be sure to ask for a trail map at park headquarters—the Big Creek Loop Trail is not shown on the general park map.

Safety note: Alligators are prolific at Brazos Bend State Park, particularly around New Horseshoe Lake. They can come as close as 5 feet away, with no fence or barrier separating you from them,

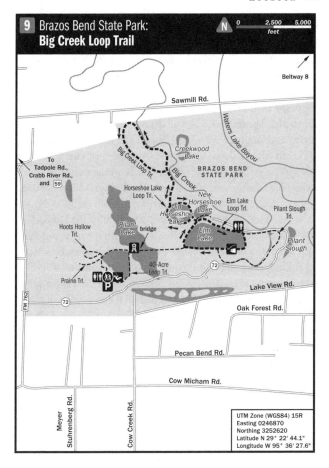

so pay close attention to your surroundings and do not let small children run ahead of you. Most of these alligators are used to people, but always err on the side of caution. Do not let pets drink from the lake or enter the water under any circumstances (water stations are along the trails for both people and dogs). In addition, watch out for snakes, some of which are poisonous.

■ UP CLOSE

Park in the last lot heading toward New Horseshoe Lake, and go left out of the lot toward a FISHING UP AHEAD sign; then go right to a concrete walkway. Continue past a trailhead sign for the Horseshoe Lake Loop on the right, and get on a gravel trail, hiking past a bench on the left and a sign on the right describing the canebrake. The trail is wide, well defined, and heavily used in the spring and summer. New Horseshoe Lake is on your right and Old Horseshoe Lake is on your left. Continue past a bench on the left and curve left. Go by another bench on the right that overlooks New Horseshoe Lake. Go straight through an intersection, where a trail joins from the left, and pass a bench on the right.

At a fork, bear right and hike past a sign for the Horseshoe Lake Loop Trail, on the right. Pass a bench on the right and then bear left at the next fork. While hiking past the water, be watchful for alligators sunning themselves on the banks at all times. Also be aware of banana spiders from spring to late fall on some parts of the trail. Most of them are high in the trees, allowing you to duck under their webs. Other wildlife you may see includes bobcats, coyotes, raccoons, gray and red foxes, river otters, feral hogs, white-tailed deer, and rodents. About 21 species of reptiles and amphibians are found here, including American alligators, snakes (some poisonous), turtles, lizards, and frogs. Brazos Bend State Park is also home to 290 species of birds, such as migratory waterfowl, shorebirds, wading birds, songbirds, and raptors.

The vegetation on the left side of the trail is thick; to the right, along the lakeshore, is riparian vegetation. Follow the trail as it bends right and then passes a bench on the right. The area on the left opens up considerably, with the trail curving right again, past a bench on the right. The dirt trail follows the contour of the lake; as you move farther from the lake, the trailside vegetation closes in and the trail surface changes to grass and dirt. Soon you pass a sign for the Big Creek Loop Trail on the left. At a fork, bear left to get on the Big Creek Loop Trail and head into the woods. The trail, hemmed in by foliage, is nevertheless easy to follow. To the left are a clearing and a very old oak tree whose limbs overarch the trail.

The trail takes a big leftward bend, giving you a fine view of Big Creek on your right. A steep slope beside Big Creek can be slippery and conceal poisonous snakes, so stay on the trail at all times. The trail curves right, now atop the creek bank. Follow the trail as it winds toward a spillway for the creek. Cross the spillway and go past a bench on the right that overlooks Big Creek; then continue past a small pond on the left. At the next Big Creek Loop Trail sign, go straight, keeping the creek on your right. A large open field is on your left. The trail heads uphill, bending left. Here the vegetation is denser and the trail surface is predominantly grass, but still easy to follow.

Continue as the trail bends left under a canopy of trees. The creek is on your right and a large clearing on your left. As the trail bends right, go past trail markers hanging in the trees on the left. Near a state-park boundary sign on a fence ahead, the trail bends left and passes under some trees. At an upcoming fork, bear left; a barrier prevents you from going straight. This part of the trail is very grassy and can be muddy or overgrown due to lack of use. The area on the right is low and can be under water, so stay on the trail.

Once out of the trees, the trail wanders through a large clearing. Where it bends left, you can see the elevated trail on which you hiked before getting on this loop. Go left toward another Big Creek Loop Trail sign, and then go right to get back on the elevated trail. Now Big Creek is on your left as you clamber up the creek bank. At the end of the Big Creek Loop Trail, take the left fork to get back on the Horseshoe Lake Loop Trail. The trail heads downhill and left, with New Horseshoe Lake on your right. A low marsh is on your left, and a short viewing platform is on the right. Go past a bench and a wetlands, both left.

Hike on the now-grassy trail past a bench on the left and another on the right. Look left for a small lake through the trees. The trail heads uphill and left, with water on both sides. At the next intersection, go straight and slightly left toward Elm Lake, which is ahead. At the intersection beyond, go left and continue to the parking lot.

■ TO THE TRAILHEAD

From Beltway 8 and US 59, head west 10.75 miles on US 59 and exit at Crabb River Road. Turn left, go 8.69 miles to Tadpole Road, and turn left. Go 5.7 miles to the entrance of the park on the left. The parking lot is at the north end of the park, past the nature center and Elm Lake.

Galveston Island State Park Trails

■ OVERVIEW

LENGTH: 4.3 miles	**WHEELCHAIR ACCESS:** No
CONFIGURATION: Loops	**FACILITIES:** Restrooms at park headquarters, parking, campsites, nature center, picnic tables
SCENERY: Bay marshes, bayous, coastal prairie, tidal wetlands, ponds	
EXPOSURE: Sunny	**SPECIAL COMMENTS:** Alligators and poisonous snakes are in the park, so stay on the trail at all times. The coastal grasses beside the trail are dense and provide good protection for these snakes. Before starting your hike, you must pay an entrance fee at park headquarters, on the other side of Seawall Boulevard (FM 3005).
TRAIL TRAFFIC: Light	
TRAIL SURFACE: Sand and grass	
HIKING TIME: 2 hours	
DRIVING DISTANCE: 33 miles from the intersection of Beltway 8 and I-45	
ACCESS: $5 per person age 13 and older; open 8 a.m.–10 p.m.	**MORE INFORMATION:** (409) 737-1222, tpwd.state.tx.us/spdest/findadest/parks/galveston
MAPS: USGS Lake Como; trail maps available at park headquarters and at the Web site below (click "Map of Park" at left)	

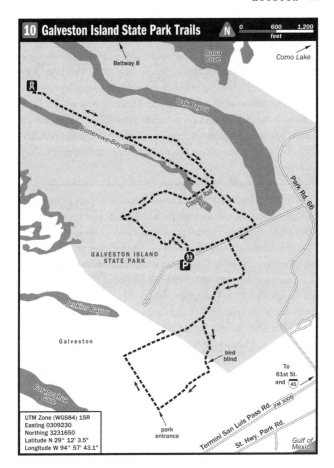

10 Galveston Island State Park Trails

Beltway 8
Dana Cove
Como Lake
Oak Bayou
Butterowe Bayou
Clapper Rail Trl.
GALVESTON ISLAND STATE PARK
Jenkins Bayou
Galveston
Carancahua Cove
bird blind
To 61st St. and 45
park entrance
Termini San Luis Pass Rd. FM 3005
St. Hwy. Park Rd.
Gulf of Mexico
Park Rd. 66

0 600 1,200
feet

UTM Zone (WGS84) 15R
Easting 0309230
Northing 3231650
Latitude N 29° 12' 3.5"
Longitude W 94° 57' 43.1"

■ SNAPSHOT

Galveston Island State Park is on the west end of Galveston Island and encompasses slightly more than 2,000 acres. The site was acquired by the state in 1969 from private owners under the State Parks Bond Program and was opened to the public in 1975. The park offers camping, bird-watching, nature study, hiking, cycling, fishing, beach access, and swimming.

Like the rest of Galveston Island, the park sustained major damage from Hurricane Ike in September 2008. The West Bay side, where the hiking trails are found, emerged relatively unscathed (most of the damage was concentrated on the Gulf of Mexico side). The park reopened in June 2009; hiking, beach access, and other amenities have been restored, but the rebuilding is expected to continue for another three to five years.

■ UP CLOSE

To start the hike, head toward white posts to get on a grass trail and go north toward an observation tower. The trail is about 6 feet wide, with low coastal grasses and shrubs growing on both sides. Continue toward the observation platform and climb the steps for a great view of the bay, marshes, and wetlands of Galveston. Once off the platform, head left (west) of the platform and pass a sign about the Galveston Bay Marsh. Go left at the sign to get back on the grass trail. At a fork, bear right on a sandy trail.

Galveston Island State Park is home to hundreds of species of birds, including pelicans, hummingbirds, herons, egrets, owls, spoonbills, ducks, geese, hawks, and eagles. You may also see coyotes, raccoons, armadillos, marsh rabbits, snakes, and alligators. And if you fish, try your luck for spotted sea trout, croaker, redfish, black drum, flounder, and sand trout. The park is 1 foot above sea level, making for very flat terrain. Vegetation less than 1 foot high borders the trail, allowing you to see for miles in all directions. Standing on the trail, you can see Jenkins Bayou to your left and houses just beyond the bayou. Crab holes dot the ground all along the sandy trail, indicating that this is a good area for catching blue crab, calico crab, and fiddler crab. At a fork, bear right and get on a much wider trail. Go to the next intersection, where a trail joins on the right, and follow the trail as it curves right. As you leave the marsh, the trail narrows and trailside grasses increase. Look left for Carancahua Cove in the distance.

Continue as the trail heads slightly uphill and changes to a grassy surface. Vegetation beside the trail here includes prickly pear cacti, mesquite and other shrubs, and coastal grasses. At the next intersection, go left on the Clapper Rail Trail, a long bridge over the Butterowe Bayou. Once off the rail trail, the trail surface changes to shells and sand. At the next intersection, bear left and get back on a grass trail. Butterowe Bayou is now on your left. Where the trail heads downhill, it may be slippery when wet, so watch your footing. Look right for houses around Como Lake. Go through the next intersection, where a trail joins on the right. Now head past a bench and toward another observation tower.

Stay left of the bayou and go past two benches on the left. Sand and low vegetation may make the trail difficult to see; continue to head toward the observation tower. Look left for Texas City and the Galveston Causeway Bridge on a clear day.

From the observation tower, turn around and retrace your route to the first double path you come to. Take the path on the left, as the one on the right is the trail you were on earlier. The trail surface changes back to grass as you leave the marsh, and vegetation increases on both sides. Go by two benches on the right before the trail curves right. Continue through the next intersection, with the trail you hiked earlier on your right. At the next intersection, bear right, toward the Clapper Rail Trail. Just before the rail trail, bear left onto a grass-covered trail. As you head toward the park road, Oak Bayou is now on your left, along with camping and picnic facilities. At the park road, turn right and hike to a trailhead on the left. At the trailhead, go left to get back on a wide, grassy trail. At a fork, bear left, toward FM 3005, which is south (left) of the trail.

Continue past a fishing pond on your left as the trail heads uphill. Go straight through an intersection, past an observation blind on the right. At a stand of trees, head right as the trail curves and continue through the next intersection. FM 3005 is now on your left and a small pond is on the right. At a fork, go left. Continue through the next intersection and past another observation blind, on the right. At the next intersection, turn right to get on a park road that leads past a grassy parking lot. A pond is on your right, and the parking lot is on your left. Go through the next intersection, where a trail joins on the right, and pass a fenced area on your left. At the next intersection, turn right and pass a cattail pond. Continue through the next intersection, where a trail joins on the right, and retrace your route to get on the last loop. At the park road, turn left to return to the parking lot.

Note: Try to hike these trails during the cooler months, as there is no protection from the sun—the heat and mosquitoes are oppressive during the summer. Pets must be on a leash at all times. Fishing is allowed in the bayou, but you must have a valid fishing license and observe all state-park fishing rules. For a full list of the rules, check at park headquarters or go to the Web site at the beginning of this profile (click "Fishing Tip Sheet for Galveston Island State Park").

■ TO THE TRAILHEAD

From the intersection of Beltway 8 and I-45, head south 32.26 miles on I-45, exit at 61st Street, and turn right. Go 1.65 miles to Seawall Boulevard (FM 3005) and turn right. Go 9 miles to the entrance of the state park, on the left. After paying the entrance fee, turn around and go back to FM 3005. Cross FM 3005 to enter the park on the north side. Take the first left and park in the first parking lot on the right.

■ MORE FUN

Nearby attractions include **Moody Gardens** (**moodygardens.com**), which comprises an aquarium, IMAX theater, rain-forest pyramid, and private beach; the **Lone Star Flight Museum** (**lsfm.org**); **Schlitterbahn** water park (**schlitterbahn.com/gal**); the **Strand Historic District; Seawolf Park** (**galveston.com/seawolfpark**); nine historic homes and buildings; and the **Galveston Railroad Museum** (**galveston rrmuseum.com**).

■ OVERVIEW

LENGTH: 3.2 miles	**WHEELCHAIR ACCESS:** No
CONFIGURATION: Loop	**FACILITIES:** Restrooms, bathhouse, nature center, parking, picnic areas, camping, fishing piers, bike trails, park store, boat rentals, playground
SCENERY: Woodlands, marsh, lake	
EXPOSURE: Shady	
TRAIL TRAFFIC: Light weekdays, moderate weekends	**SPECIAL COMMENTS:** Watch out for bikers because the terrain is hilly and the trail is narrow. Keep an eye out for alligators and poisonous snakes; stay on the trail at all times. Pets must be leashed. Boating on the lake is restricted to boats under 19 feet long, and water skiing is prohibited. Drinking water is unavailable on the trails.
TRAIL SURFACE: Dirt and sand	
HIKING TIME: 1.5 hours	
DRIVING DISTANCE: 49 miles from the intersection of Beltway 8 and I-45	
ACCESS: $4 per person age 13 and older, or buy a yearly Texas State Parks Pass (tpwd.state.tx.us/parkpass); open 8 a.m.–10 p.m.	**MORE INFORMATION:** (936) 295-5644, tpwd.state.tx.us/spdest/findadest/parks/huntsville
MAPS: USGS Huntsville and Moore Grove; trail maps available	

■ SNAPSHOT

Huntsville State Park is a 2,083-acre recreational area near the western edge of the Southern Pine Belt. It was opened in 1938 but closed in 1940 after a flood caused the dam spillway to collapse. Officially reopened to the public in 1956, the park adjoins the Sam Houston National Forest and encloses Lake Raven. White-tailed deer, raccoons, opossums, armadillos, migratory waterfowl, and fox squirrels are just some of the wildlife found in the area. Plant life includes oaks, loblolly and shortleaf pines, and various shrubs. The Dogwood Trail hike is short and easy for most hikers, but because the elevation varies, it may be a challenge for those with limited physical abilities, such as small children and seniors.

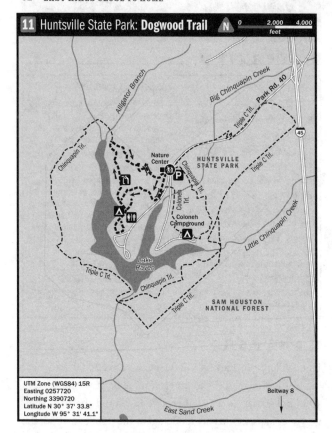

11 Huntsville State Park: **Dogwood Trail**   N   0   2,000   4,000   feet

HUNTSVILLE STATE PARK

Big Chinquapin Creek

Park Rd. 40

Triple C Trl.

45

Alligator Branch

Chinquapin Trl.

Nature Center

Chinquapin Trl.

Coloneh Trl.

Coloneh Campground

Little Chinquapin Creek

Triple C Trl.

Lake Raven

Triple C Trl.

Chinquapin Trl.

Triple C Trl.

SAM HOUSTON NATIONAL FOREST

UTM Zone (WGS84) 15R
Easting 0257720
Northing 3390720
Latitude N 30° 37' 33.8"
Longitude W 95° 31' 41.1"

Beltway 8

East Sand Creek

■ UP CLOSE

This hike includes parts of the Dogwood, Prairie Branch, and Chinquapin trails. Start at the trailhead to the left of the nature center, just inside the park. Here you'll find restrooms, parking, picnic tables, and water fountains. Head toward the Dogwood Trail sign and go left to start the hike. The trail surface is mostly dirt with old pieces of asphalt. The park road is on your left, with dense woodlands on your right. Hike across an access road and go straight to get back on the trail. The vegetation here consists of tall loblolly pines, oaks, and thick shrubs such as elderberry and holly.

The trail winds steeply downhill. Continue past a bench on the left as the trail zigzags toward the park road. Go past some parking spaces, left, before crossing a bridge marked "20." Once off the bridge, the trail heads uphill. Continue through an intersection, and look ahead for Lake Raven in the distance through the trees. Take a right fork to stay on the Dogwood Trail. A trail sign ahead is for hikers coming the other way. The trail heads uphill and away from the road, narrowing to only about 4 feet wide. A large clearing with many fallen trees—evidence of storms such as Hurricane Rita—is to the right.

Cross a service road and go straight to stay on the trail. Especially from late spring to early fall, be aware of spiderwebs across the trail and try to hike under them. Continue across another service road, heading straight and downhill. Loose rocks are here: be careful and walk slowly until the trail levels.

Parts of the trail have been washed out, and the center of it is a good foot below the sides. Either hike down the middle or hike on either side of the recessed area. The trail continues downhill, with a peek at Lake Raven up ahead. The trail narrows to about a foot wide and then widens again as you reach an intersection. Take the left fork going downhill. Campsites are now visible on your right, with restrooms and a playground up ahead. These are the last available restrooms until the end of the hike. At a HIKE AND BIKE TRAIL sign on your left, turn around and retrace to the previous intersection. Now bear left and then immediately right to get on the signed Prairie Branch Trail. The ascending trail has exposed tree roots, so be careful and watch your footing. This wide (5-plus feet) dirt trail heads away from the campgrounds and back into the woods. Pass a viewing stand on the left and head downhill as the trail bends left. As you go by a trail marker on your left, the trail heads downhill and left. Roller-coaster past several more trail markers. Look to your left for a marsh through the trees. At the signed Chinquapin Trail, bear right and then wind uphill. Go straight at an intersection marked by a HIKING TRAIL sign. The trail descends steeply to a bridge, then ascends just beyond. Continue across an access road and past a viewing stand on your right. Cross a service road and go slightly right to get back on the trail. The trail heads uphill slightly before you come to the end of the hike and the nature center. When you see the trail map on the left, go right to get to the parking lot.

■ TO THE TRAILHEAD

From the intersection of Beltway 8 and I-45, head north on I-45 49 miles to Park Road 40 and turn left. The park entrance is approximately 2 miles ahead. Park on the right just past the park entrance at the Nature Center.

■ MORE FUN

Nearby attractions include the Sam Houston Memorial Museum (samhouston.org), the Texas Prison Museum (txprisonmuseum.org), the H.E.A.R.T.S. Veterans Museum (heartsmuseum.com), Sam Houston National Forest, and Lake Conroe.

12 Lake Livingston State Park: Lake Trail

■ OVERVIEW

LENGTH: 4 miles

CONFIGURATION: Out-and-back

SCENERY: Lake Livingston, piney woods, campsites

EXPOSURE: Shady

TRAIL TRAFFIC: Light

TRAIL SURFACE: Dirt with some crushed granite

HIKING TIME: 2 hours

DRIVING DISTANCE: 55 miles from intersection of Beltway 8 and US 59

ACCESS: $3 per person age 13 and older, or buy a yearly Texas State Parks Pass (tpwd.state.tx.us/parkpass); open 8 a.m.–10 p.m.

MAPS: USGS Blanchard; trail maps available at park headquarters

WHEELCHAIR ACCESS: No

FACILITIES: Restrooms, camping, picnicking, swimming, boating, fishing, park store, showers, trail signs, horseback riding

SPECIAL COMMENTS: This hike offers the best views of the lake. Though you do pass through some campsites, you probably won't encounter many campers during the week. A fishing license is required for anyone under the age of 17. Pets must be leashed at all times.

MORE INFORMATION: (936) 365-2201, tpwd.state.tx.us/spdest/findadest/parks/lake_livingston

■ SNAPSHOT

Along an 84,800-acre reservoir, amid pine–oak woodlands, are the 635.5 acres of Lake Livingston State Park. The trails are well maintained and easy to hike, with a variety of views. The hike featured here is the only one in the park that takes you along the shores of Lake Livingston. The park also offers camping, picnicking, swimming, mountain biking, horseback riding, and boating. Boat ramps and fishing piers provide easy access to the lake, where you can catch largemouth, white, and striped bass or flathead, channel, and blue catfish. A 30-foot observation tower, near the park store and boat ramp, offers views of the park and the lake. Among the wildlife you're likely to see are white-tailed deer, raccoons, mallard ducks, swamp rabbits, armadillos, and squirrels. Lake Livingston is most crowded on weekends in the fall and spring.

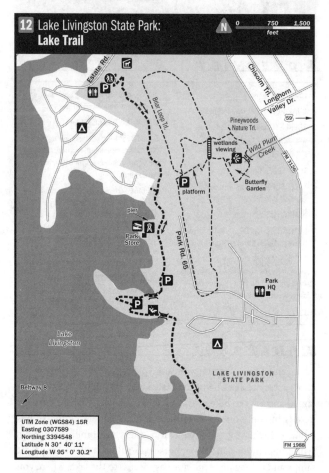

12 Lake Livingston State Park:
Lake Trail

N   0   750   1,500
        feet

UTM Zone (WGS84) 15R
Easting 0307589
Northing 3394548
Latitude N 30° 40' 11"
Longitude W 95° 0' 30.2"

■ UP CLOSE

Start the hike on the trailhead left of the restrooms. Once on
the trail, go straight, passing by campsites on your right. The
trail surface is dirt with leaves, pine needles, and some horse
manure. Even though this is not designated as an equestrian

trail, it is obviously used by horses, so watch your step. After heavy rains you may encounter standing water on this part of the trail, but there is room on both sides to go around it. Go left, away from the campsites and the parking lot. Now the trail becomes more defined and easier to follow.

The vegetation, which includes numerous downed trees from recent storms, is relatively sparse, allowing you to see deeply into the woods and the campsites just past them. Cross a paved road and soon come to an intersection. Go straight to stay on the tree-canopied trail. You can now see glimpses of the lake to your right. After the trail bends left, you can clearly see the lake on the right, with picnic tables on a point jutting out into Lake Livingston. The ground slopes steeply downhill toward the lake, so make sure you stay on the trail.

Cross a road and pick up the trail on the other side. Picnic sites are on both sides of the trail now, with the lake in full view. If you hike during the week, most of the picnic tables and campsites will be unoccupied, making for a quiet hike. Cross another road and go straight over culverts to get back on the trail. Parking is on your left, and on your right are fishing piers, an observation tower, and a park store with restrooms. Veer slightly right toward the park store. Just left of the store, go left to get back on the trail. Campsites are on your left now, with picnic tables and the lake still on your right. Go through the next intersection and head straight. The trail surface is now crushed granite with some dirt and sand. A parking lot and boat launch are down the hill at right. Continue straight across the boat-launch road, and then head slightly left to stay on the trail.

Hike past more picnic tables and go straight toward a bridge on the right. The trail heads steeply downhill to the bridge, so watch your footing. Cross the bridge over a small inlet and go right to stay on the trail. Head left and uphill, past a swimming pool on the right. Continue across the swimming pool walkway and toward yellow motorized-vehicle barriers. Go through the barriers and toward two picnic tables out on a point in the lake. At the tables, turn around and bear left and back into the trees to get back on the trail. This part of the trail runs parallel to the trail you just used. It is about 10 feet wide and continues through another set of traffic barriers. At the barriers, go right to head toward the lake. A parking lot is to your left. Before you get to the water, go left as you hike on an embankment above the water's edge.

Continue through the trees, with the lake on your immediate right and the road to your left. Pass another small inlet, right, with a bridge that has been damaged and is currently unsafe to cross. Continue straight, with a playground on your left and the trees to your right. At an intersection, turn right to get back on the trail. More campsites are on your left, and the lake is far to the right. The trail widens and goes left, past picnic tables on both sides of the trail. Restrooms with showers are on the right through the trees. Continue across a road and then left as the trail curves away from the lake. Avoid the numerous paths made by campers on both sides of the trail. Continue straight, past another set of restrooms on the left. As the trail swings left, the lake is no longer visible. Continue just past some benches and a nature-trail sign on the right. The nature trail is a little over 0.6 miles long but currently has a bridge out, so go straight to the other end of the trail and turn around. Now retrace your route to the parking area.

■ TO THE TRAILHEAD

From Beltway 8 and US 59, head north on US 59 for 51 miles and turn left onto FM 1988. Drive 4 miles to FM 3126 and turn right. Drive 0.5 miles to Park Road 65 and turn left. To get to the Lake Trail trailhead, take Park Road 65 to the first intersection and turn right. At the end of the road, turn left and park in the lot, to the left of the restrooms.

■ MORE FUN

Lake Livingston is near the ghost town of Swartwout, the meeting place of Polk County's first commissioner's court before Livingston was selected as the county seat. Swartwout was also a steamboat landing on the Trinity River in the 1830s and 1850s. The City of Livingston is only 10 miles from the park, providing all the amenities and conveniences of a small town. Hundreds of privately owned parks and marinas are in the area around Lake Livingston, providing access to the lake.

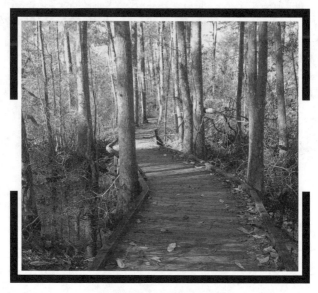

A boardwalk on the Kirby Nature Trail

Outlying Hikes

■ OVERVIEW

LENGTH: 1.2 miles	**WHEELCHAIR ACCESS:** No
CONFIGURATION: Loop	**FACILITIES:** Restrooms, Discovery Center, parking, picnic areas, fishing piers
SCENERY: Slough, marshes, prairies, woodlands	**SPECIAL COMMENTS:** A picnic area and restrooms are available at the Discovery Center, but there is no water, so bring your own along with sunscreen, mosquito repellent, and a hat. Poisonous snakes and alligators lurk in the refuge, so be cautious at all times and don't let young children run ahead of you.
EXPOSURE: Sunny	
TRAIL TRAFFIC: Light	
TRAIL SURFACE: Grass	
HIKING TIME: 1 hour	
DRIVING DISTANCE: 52 miles from the intersection of Beltway 8 and I-288	
ACCESS: Free; daily, sunrise–sunset	**MORE INFORMATION:** (979) 922-1037, fws.gov/refuges
MAPS: USGS Oyster Creek; trail signs and trail map	

■ SNAPSHOT

Brazoria National Wildlife Refuge, which opened in the late 1980s, is home to more than 400 species of wildlife. Its marshes and prairies create some of the richest environments on Earth. Two hunting areas exist—the Christmas Point Public Waterfowl Hunting Area and the Middle Bayou Public Waterfowl Hunting area; check with headquarters for restrictions and seasons. You can pier-fish at Bastrop Bayou (the pier is handicap accessible) or bank-fish at Clay Banks and Salt Lake.

■ UP CLOSE

The Big Slough Trail is named after a freshwater lifeline that runs through the prairie, marsh, and woodland habitats. Start the hike in the Discovery Center parking lot. Hike toward the marsh and boardwalk behind the building, passing under the picnic

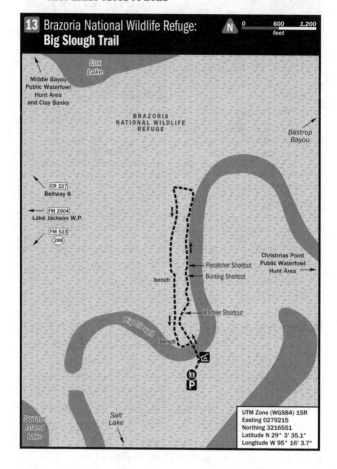

13 Brazoria National Wildlife Refuge:
Big Slough Trail

N

0   600   1,200
feet

Cox Lake

Middle Bayou
Public Waterfowl
Hunt Area
and Clay Banks

BRAZORIA
NATIONAL WILDLIFE
REFUGE

Bastrop
Bayou

CR 227
Beltway 8

FM 2004
Lake Jackson W.P.

FM 523
288

Christmas Point
Public Waterfowl
Hunt Area

Flycatcher Shortcut

Bunting Shortcut

bench

Warbler Shortcut

Big Slough

bench

P

Square
Island
Lake

Salt
Lake

UTM Zone (WGS84) 15R
Easting 0279215
Northing 3216551
Latitude N 29° 3' 35.1"
Longitude W 95° 16' 3.7"

pavilion. Once on the boardwalk, go to the right past some newly constructed pylons on the left. A sign on the right describes the butterfly habitat just off the slough. The boardwalk is several feet above the water and a safe distance from any alligators. Follow the boardwalk as it wanders over the slough. Stop to see how many ducks, snakes, and alligators you can spot. Continue under another pavilion with benches and past a nature sign about the coastal wetlands on the right. Pass a platform on the right that takes you closer to the water and the wildlife.

Continue along the boardwalk past a sign about the American alligator, and then get off the boardwalk heading to the right. Go by a bench on the left as the trail surface changes to grass. Follow a trail sign for the Big Slough Trail and pass Trail Marker 1. These markers coincide with the information in the Big Slough Trail Guide, which you can pick up at the information center. Some of the plants on this trail include grasses, sedges, rushes, cattails, water lilies, palmettos, prickly pear cacti, ash trees, Chinese tallow trees, yaupon bushes, and willows. Continue past Trail Marker 2, where the vegetation on both sides of the trail is thick and impenetrable. Pass a nature sign on the right about songbirds—neotropical migrants that include kingbirds, yellow warblers, gray catbirds, and common yellowthroats. As the trail heads right and into the trees, watch where you step, as this trail is frequently used by cows. The slightly elevated trail curves right and then passes the Warbler Shortcut, which joins from the left. Continue straight, passing a sign about the wildlife signs, which include tracks, feathers, and scat.

Wildlife you may see includes coyotes, bobcats, raccoons, opossums, swamp rabbits, skunks, armadillos, feral hogs, alligators, and snakes, both poisonous (eastern cottonmouth and rattlesnake) and nonpoisonous (rat and water snakes). Continue past Trail Marker 3 and then curve right. Now swing left, past Trail Marker 4 and then through the intersection with the Bunting Shortcut. The route then veers left past a bench on the left and goes through the intersection with the Flycatcher Shortcut. Go straight to find Trail Marker 5; then swing left to Trail Marker 6.

The wide trail passes Trail Marker 7 and then winds to Trail Marker 8. Now head uphill, past Trail Marker 9 and a viewing platform on the right. A bench on the platform overlooks a small marsh. Continue as the trail bends left; to the right is an off-limits section of the refuge. Follow the sign for the Big Slough Trail, hiking left and uphill. Look to your right for a large stand of trees in the distance, past the coastal prairie. Throughout the hike, look for refuge birds such as great blue herons, moorhens, northern cardinals, mockingbirds, quail, snow geese, roseate spoonbills, and black-necked stilts.

Continue past Trail Markers 10, 11, and 12, and through an intersection with a trail on the left. The refuge-boundary fence is now on your right, just beyond the vegetation. After Trail Marker 13, the trail bends left and then takes a quick turn right. Continue past a bench on the left and an intersection with a trail on the left. Go past Trail Marker 14. A stand of trees on the right includes the Osage orange and the sugar hackberry. Wander back and forth to the next intersection, with a trail on the left, and then follow the trail-exit sign. The boundary fence is still on your right as you pass a bench on the left.

After Trail Marker 15, the trail climbs slightly uphill and curves left. You can see the Discovery Center straight ahead, past a small lily pond. Curve left, keeping the pond on your right. You are headed back to the boardwalk and the Big Slough. At the board-walk, head to the right and retrace your route to the trailhead.

■ TO THE TRAILHEAD

From Beltway 8 and I-288, head south 38 miles to FM 2004 and take a left. Go 6.3 miles to FM 523 and turn right. Drive 5.6 miles to County Road 227 and turn left, driving 2 miles to the entrance of the refuge, on the right. The Discovery Center is 3 miles ahead.

■ MORE FUN

Lake Jackson Wilderness Park (page 93), the Gulf Coast Bird Observatory (gcbo.org), and San Bernard National Wildlife Refuge (fws.gov/refuges) are less than 15 miles from Brazoria National Wildlife Refuge. Brazos Bend State Park (page 52) and George Ranch Historical Park (georgeranch.org), a living-history site and working cattle ranch, are also close by.

Armand Bayou Nature Center: Martyn and Karankawa Trails

■ OVERVIEW

LENGTH: 2.9 miles

CONFIGURATION: 2 loops

SCENERY: Creek beds, woodlands, bayou, wetlands, boardwalk

EXPOSURE: Shady

TRAIL TRAFFIC: Light

TRAIL SURFACE: Dirt

HIKING TIME: 2 hours

DRIVING DISTANCE: 12 miles from the junction of Beltway 8 and I-45

ACCESS: $3 per person age 18 and older; $1 children ages 5–17 and seniors age 60 and older; open Tu–Sa, 9 a.m.–5 p.m., Su, noon–5.

MAPS: USGS League City; trail maps available on-site and at abnc.org/uploads/pdf/ABNC-Trail-Map.pdf

WHEELCHAIR ACCESS: No

FACILITIES: Restrooms, picnic tables, interpretive center, tours, trail signs

SPECIAL COMMENTS: Bikes and pets are not allowed on the hiking trails at any time. Bring plenty of bug repellent, even in cool weather.

MORE INFORMATION: (281) 474-2551, abnc.org

■ SNAPSHOT

The Armand Bayou Nature Center comprises three different ecosystems: bayou, forest, and tallgrass prairie. It has been designated as one of only four Texas Coastal Preserves and is one of the largest bayous in the Houston area that is not channeled. In addition to hiking trails, the center features a raptor house; the 1895 Hanson Farm House, with a garden, barn, windmill, and pond; pontoon-boat rides; and canoe rides by reservation. The Martyn and Karankawa trails run parallel to each other, but they are very different. The Martyn Trail is narrower and goes into deeper woods, whereas the Karankawa Trail runs along the edge of a bayou. Combined, they make a fine hike of almost 3 miles, with helpful signage and rest benches along the way.

■ UP CLOSE

To start the Martyn and Karankawa trails, park in the first lot on the left as you enter the nature center. Go to the information

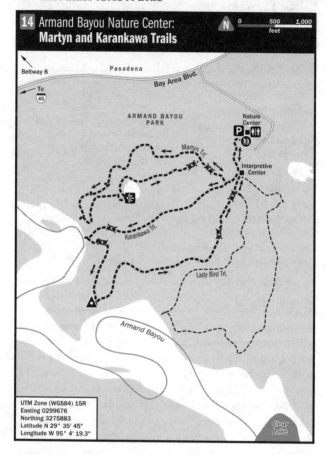

14 Armand Bayou Nature Center:
Martyn and Karankawa Trails

N

0   500   1,000
feet

Beltway 8

Pasadena

Bay Area Blvd.

To
45

ARMAND BAYOU
PARK

Nature
Center

Martyn Trl.

Interpretive
Center

Karankawa Trl.

Lady Bird Trl.

Armand Bayou

Clear
Lake

UTM Zone (WGS84) 15R
Easting 0299676
Northing 3275883
Latitude N 29° 35' 45"
Longitude W 95° 4' 19.3"

center just across the parking lot to pay the entry fee and pick up a trail map. Go left out of the building, past the raptor cage, and down the boardwalk. Signs warn that the boardwalk is slippery when wet, so use caution. Continue past benches and nature signs along the extensive boardwalk, which crosses wetlands. More than 370 species of birds, mammals, amphibians, and reptiles inhabit this 2,500-acre wildlife and nature preserve, including white-tailed deer, armadillos, bobcats, coyotes, swamp rabbits, turtles, alligators, and snakes (both poisonous and nonpoisonous). The bird population comprises more than 220 species, including warblers, flycatchers, orioles, painted buntings, ospreys, owls, kites, and hawks.

Just before the boardwalk ends, note the sign warning about poison ivy. Some of the other plants found in the preserve are yaupon, Spanish moss, white oak, black gum, ironwood, American beautyberry, and wax myrtle. Once off the boardwalk, go to the interpretive center straight ahead. A trail sign and map are just past the center. The trailhead is just past an observation blind on the right. The trail, about 9 feet wide here, is dirt with some shale. Continue along the trail until you come to the first set of trail markers. Here turn right to get on the Martyn Trail. Cross a bridge and curve right as the trail narrows to about 6 feet wide. Notice the predominance of lichen on the trail, indicating that the preserve stays fairly wet and the trails are not heavily used.

Follow a curvy course past a bench on the right. A high tree canopy shades the mostly level trail. Because of standing water during certain times of the year, little vegetation is on the forest floor. Cross another bridge and then, at the Martyn Trail sign, turn right. Pass beneath a naturally growing arbor, and then walk past a bench on the right. As the trail turns slightly right, hike under another low arbor. Now holly trees and white oaks line the route. Go past another Martyn Trail sign on the left. Look right for Armand Bayou through the trees.

Hike past another Martyn Trail sign and then bear right at a fork to follow a spur trail to a bayou overlook. At the end of the spur are benches and a nature sign describing the Galveston Bay Marsh, one of the most diverse habitats in the Houston area. The marsh is an estuary, one of Earth's most productive and important ecosystems. Estuaries are "nature's nurseries," nurturing juvenile shrimp, oysters, crabs, and finfish. Without these habitats, fish populations would decline dramatically. After enjoying the view, retrace to the Martyn Trail sign and turn right. The trail heads slightly uphill and then winds through trees. Go straight through the next intersection, where a trail joins on the right. At the next trail marker, take the Martyn Trail to the left. The vegetation under the trees contains more tall grasses and low bushes, indicating that this area is not periodically covered in water, in contrast with the previous section of the trail. Continue past the next trail marker and then go right to stay on the Martyn Trail. Turn right at the intersection and take a short spur to a wildlife-observation platform. After visiting the platform, retrace to the previous intersection and then bear right. Keep right, past numerous oak trees that regularly drop acorns on the trail, creating a bit of an uneven surface. Continue straight past a hiking sign and then follow the trail to the right, under a tree that leans over the trail.

Just past a bench on the left, the trail surface again becomes grassy, making it a little more difficult to see. Once the trail curves left and then past a bench, it widens and is much more visible. The trail winds to a bridge, which you cross. At the next intersection, go right, following a sign that reads TO RETURN. Go back over the bridge you crossed at the beginning of the hike and then, at an intersection, turn right to get on the Karankawa Trail. The wide dirt trail passes an area without much vegetation on the forest floor, indicating periodic flooding. Hike past a barbed-wire fence on your left, continuing through the trees and past a bench on the left. Cross a bridge and then go past a clearing on the left with a picnic table; a trail marker is on the right. Go straight to reach a small pier that juts into the bayou. A small fishing shack and some benches sit atop the pier. Turn around and retrace to the previous intersection; then bear right to get back on the Karankawa Trail. Cross a wide bridge over a deep creek and follow the twisty trail past a bench on the right. At a bayou-overlook sign, turn right on a spur trail to visit the overlook, where you'll find benches for wildlife viewing. Now retrace along the spur to the previous intersection, and turn right to regain the Karankawa Trail. Go past a bench on the left and then a trail marker on the right. Pass several benches and cross a small bridge. At the next trail marker, go left and then over another small bridge. Cross a third bridge before reaching the interpretive center. Go around the interpretive center to get back on the boardwalk. Follow the boardwalk back to the parking lot and the end of the hike.

■ TO THE TRAILHEAD

From Beltway 8 and I-45, head south 6 miles on I-45 and exit at Bay Area Boulevard. Turn left and go 6 miles to the entrance of the Armand Bayou Nature Center, on the right. Park in the first parking lot on the left.

15 Big Thicket National Preserve: Kirby Nature Trail

■ OVERVIEW

LENGTH: 3.3 miles

CONFIGURATION: Balloon

SCENERY: Big thicket, woodlands, cypress swamps, creeks, sloughs, boardwalks

EXPOSURE: Shady

TRAIL TRAFFIC: Light–moderate

TRAIL SURFACE: Dirt

HIKING TIME: 1.5 hours

DRIVING DISTANCE: 102 miles from the intersection of Beltway 8 and I-10 east

ACCESS: Free; visitor center open 9 a.m.–5 p.m.

MAPS: USGS Kountze North; trail maps available

WHEELCHAIR ACCESS: No

FACILITIES: Restrooms, visitor center, parking, picnic tables, water fountains, fishing

SPECIAL COMMENTS: Try to hike in cooler weather, from late fall to late spring. Register at the trailhead before starting your hike. The preserve harbors poisonous snakes, feral hogs, and, most recently, mountain lions, so use caution and stay on the trail at all times. Pets are not allowed on the trails. Bring insect repellent, and avoid disturbing bee, wasp, or fire-ant nests.

MORE INFORMATION: (409) 951-6700, nps.gov/bith

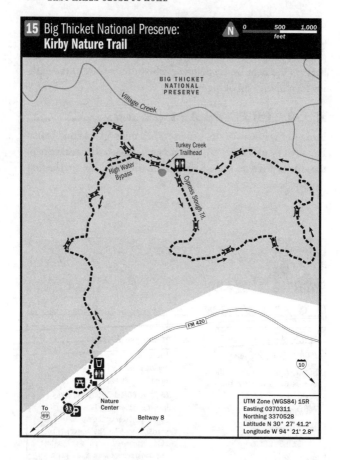

15 Big Thicket National Preserve:
Kirby Nature Trail

N　0　500　1,000
feet

BIG THICKET
NATIONAL
PRESERVE

Village Creek

Turkey Creek
Trailhead

High Water
Bypass

Cypress Slough Trl.

FM 420

10

Nature
Center

Beltway 8

To
69

UTM Zone (WGS84) 15R
Easting 0370311
Northing 3370528
Latitude N 30° 27' 41.2"
Longitude W 94° 21' 2.8"

■ SNAPSHOT

The Big Thicket was the first national preserve in the federal park system, encompassing more than 97,000 acres in nine land units. Established in 1974, it was recognized in 2001 by the American Bird Conservancy as a Globally Important Bird Area. The preserve's various ecosystems include eastern hardwood forests, Gulf coastal plains, and Midwest prairies. The resident animals include bobcats, mountain lions, armadillos, white-tailed deer, skunks, raccoons, and coyotes. You may also encounter snakes such as the coral snake (poisonous) and speckled king snake (nonpoisonous). Among the preserve's birdlife are Bachman's sparrows, yellow-billed cuckoos, wood ducks, roadrunners, pileated woodpeckers, and brown-headed nuthatches.

There are nine trails in five of the land units, ranging from 0.5 to 18 miles in length. Permits are not required for hiking, but all hikers should register at the trailhead, where detailed maps are available. Bicycles are not allowed on the Kirby Nature Trail.

■ U P   C L O S E

Start your hike at the Kirby Nature Trail parking lot and head east toward the trail sign at the east end of the lot. The trail surface is asphalt with landscaping timbers as edging. The trail curves right and then slightly left as you enter a picnic area. Continue through the picnic area on a wooden boardwalk toward the forest entrance. Water fountains, restrooms, and a small nature center are also in this area. Go past a sign on your left describing the nature trail and what you might expect to see. Head toward the trees and go through an intersection, passing restrooms on your right. Once in the forest, you'll pass a sign about the important relationship between large forests and the air we breathe. At the next intersection, go left, following a trail sign. The trail surface changes to dirt but continues to be edged by landscape timbers.

The trail curves right, past a numbered marker and a nature sign about American beech. There is considerable evidence of Hurricanes Rita and Ike, with a number of downed trees lining both sides of the trail. The trail passes magnolias, beeches, water oaks, and loblolly pines. Get on a boardwalk that crosses a cypress bog on each side of the trail. The boardwalk is slippery when wet: watch your footing at all times. As you step off the boardwalk, the trail heads slightly uphill. Continue past a nature sign about American holly. Go past a bench on the left and then a nature sign about white oak. Cross a short bridge and head left. The trail narrows to about 4 feet wide, just past nature signs about Eastern and American hornbeam. Wind past a bench on the right. Cross a boardwalk and head uphill as the trail surface changes to sand and takes a big bend left. After a straight stretch, the trail bends right and past a bench on the right. Continue to another boardwalk and past another trail marker and a nature sign for bald cypress. The boardwalk takes you over another cypress swamp. Once you get off the board-walk, the trail climbs right. Take the right fork at a trail sign to follow the High Water Bypass.

At the next intersection, go straight on the Inner Loop Trail and cross a bridge over a third cypress swamp. Get off the boardwalk, pass a bench on the left, and then head uphill and left. Passing Trail Marker 18 on the left, you walk past a bench overlooking a large pond, on the left. At an intersection, turn right to stay on the Inner Loop Trail. Pass a nature sign about sweetgum trees and Trail Marker 19. Cross a bridge and hike uphill as the trail curves left. Continue past Trail Markers 20 and 21, and a bench on the left. The trail bends right and then crosses a bridge, passing a sign about rattan vines. Beyond the bridge, the trail swings right and uphill. Go past Trail Marker 23, a sign about the water oak on the right, and a bench on the left. At an intersection, take the left fork uphill. Cross a bridge and pass a bench on the left. The trail heads uphill and left, changing to dirt and grass. Continue past a bench on the right, cross a bridge, and hike past another bench on the right as the trail heads uphill. After a sweeping rightward bend, go by a bench on the right as the trail heads uphill and left. Lichen and moss grow on the trail here, indicating that this part of the Kirby Nature Trail is used less than other parts. The trail heads downhill and past two benches, one on the left and one on the right. Cross a bridge and follow the trail as it winds past another bridge, on the left. Continue past a bench on the left and onto a short boardwalk over a cypress swamp. Once off the boardwalk, pass another bench as the trail heads uphill. The vegetation is very thick here, as you cross another bridge and hike past a bench on the right overlooking a pond, also on the right.

Go past a bench on the right as the trail winds right, past a trailhead sign for the Turkey Creek Trail. Continue straight to stay on the Kirby Nature Trail. At an intersection, head straight and then slightly right. Go past a bench overlooking a pond, both on the right. Cross a boardwalk and take the right fork to get on the Cypress Slough Trail. Cross a bridge, continuing past a bench on the left and Trail Marker 16. Cross another bridge and hike past a nature sign about water tupelo. The trail heads uphill, with a bench on the right and a bog on the left. Walk past Trail Marker 15 and then cross a bridge. Once over the bridge, hike past a bench on the left. Continue to yet another bridge over a cypress swamp, and then head uphill to Trail Marker 14. At a fork, bear right and retrace your steps. As you exit the woods, the restrooms are on your left. Continue along the wooden boardwalk to the parking lot.

■ TO THE TRAILHEAD

From the intersection of Beltway 8 and I-10, drive east 69 miles on I-10 to the Highway 69/96 North exit in Beaumont. Go 32 miles on Highway 69/96 to FM 420 and turn right. Follow signs to the visitor center, which is on the left. The trailhead for the Kirby Nature Trail is 2.5 miles east of the visitor center on FM 420.

16 Anahuac National Wildlife Refuge: Shoveler Pond Trail

■ OVERVIEW

LENGTH: 4.2 miles

CONFIGURATION: Loop

SCENERY: Bayou, wetlands, ponds, willow stands, woodlot, butterfly–hummingbird habitat, coastal marsh, coastal prairie

EXPOSURE: Sunny

TRAIL TRAFFIC: Light

TRAIL SURFACE: Dirt and gravel, some pavement and grass

HIKING TIME: 2 hours

DRIVING DISTANCE: 47.5 miles from the intersection of Beltway 8 and I-10 east

ACCESS: Free; main gate open 24 hours a day, seven days a week; public-use areas open 1 hour before sunrise–1 hour after sunset

MAPS: USGS Frozen Point

WHEELCHAIR ACCESS: Yes

FACILITIES: Visitor-information station, restrooms, gift shop, fishing, boating, canoe-and-kayak launch, parking, wildlife-viewing areas

SPECIAL COMMENTS: This is a very open trail with no shade, so it's best hiked from late fall to early spring. Pets must be leashed at all times. Bicycles are permitted on gravel roads only; all-terrain vehicles, airboats, and personal watercraft are prohibited. No drinking water is available anywhere in the refuge. Be aware at all times of snakes, alligators, fire ants, and mosquitoes.

MORE INFORMATION: (409) 267-3337, fws.gov/refuges

■ SNAPSHOT

The Shoveler Pond Trail includes the Butterfly and Hummingbird Habitat, the Willows Trail, and the Shoveler Pond Loop, which encircles a 220-acre freshwater impoundment with opportunities to view alligators, birds, and other marsh wildlife. The refuge encompasses more than 34,000 acres bordering Galveston Bay. Its bayous meander through floodplains, creating an extensive coastal marsh-and-prairie landscape. Southerly breezes from the Gulf of Mexico result in high humidity and an average rainfall of more than 51 inches. (*Anahuac* is an Aztec word meaning "watery plain"; however, there is no connection between the area and the Aztecs.) Anahuac National Wildlife Refuge is a recognized stop on the Great Texas Coastal Birding Trail.

HOUSTON **85**

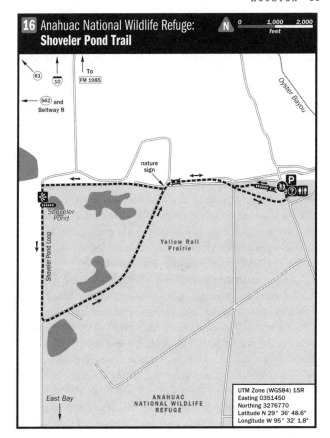

16 Anahuac National Wildlife Refuge:
Shoveler Pond Trail

■ UP CLOSE

Start the hike at the Butterfly and Hummingbird Habitat, behind
the visitor-information station (where restrooms are available).
Walk toward the flagpole to get on a paved surface that meanders through a garden built to attract hummingbirds and butterflies. At an intersection, go left. A pond is on your left, with
a bench and the garden on your right. Cross a small bridge and

then follow the trail to the right. Look left to see a large expanse of water in the distance. The prairie stretches for miles on your right. Take the next fork left, as the trail intersects tall grasses and bushes. Step onto a boardwalk to continue the hike. Pass a bench on the left and then another on the right. The boardwalk trail winds to another bench on the right overlooking a small pond. Continue through an intersection, where a trail departs left to an observation deck.

Now the boardwalk turns right past a handicapped-parking space on the left. At a fork, bear left to step off the boardwalk and onto a grass trail. Pass a bench on the right and follow the fence line on your right. A stand of willow trees and a small pond are now on your left. Stop at a nature sign to learn about the neo-tropical birds that make a 600-mile journey across the Gulf of Mexico, including the palm warbler, scissor-tailed flycatcher, and eastern kingbird. You may see more songbirds in the wooded areas and shorebirds on the mudflats and in the shallow water. As many as 27 species of ducks stop over between October and March, including green-winged teal, gadwall, northern shoveler, and northern pintail. Flocks of geese in excess of 80,000 are found in the marshes, rice fields, and mudflats. Roseate spoonbills, white-faced ibises, and great and snowy egrets are also plentiful.

Continue along the grass trail to the reserve road, and then go right to get on the Shoveler Pond Trail. This dirt-and-gravel road is easy underfoot and affords many opportunities to see ducks and other birds, alligators, snakes, and turtles. The nocturnal wildlife in the refuge includes river otters, raccoons, skunks, muskrats, opossums, and bobcats. To ensure the integrity of the habitat, the refuge employs such management tools as grazing, farming, controlled burning, exotic-plant control, shoreline stabilization, and water-level manipulation.

Continue along the road past a water channel on your left. Biking and driving are permitted on this road, so be aware of cyclists and cars coming from behind. Cross a bridge and continue past a gate on the right. The road bends left to the start of the Shoveler Pond Loop. Go right to get on the 2.5-mile trail. Water is on both sides of the trail here, with an amazing number of birds and turtles. Shoveler Pond is also home to many alligators, so be on your guard at all times: no fences are between you and them.

This is one of the most wildlife-rich hikes I have found in the Houston area, so take your time and make a list of all the mammals, reptiles, and birds you spot. Continue toward an observation platform that overlooks Shoveler Pond and provides an excellent view of the area. Once off the platform, bear left along a lengthy stretch of straight road. The terrain to your right is so flat that you can see for miles across marshes and mudflats to the eastern side of Galveston Bay. Soon you reach the Shoveler Pond boardwalk, left. A handicapped-parking space at the head of the boardwalk accommodates wheelchairs. The boardwalk takes you into the middle of Shoveler Pond, offering views that you can't see from the trail.

Once off the boardwalk, head left. Follow the trail as it bends left and past a gate on the right. Again, water is on both sides of the trail as you head back toward the visitor-information station. At an intersection, continue straight over some culverts and a small channel of water. Look to your left for the Shoveler Pond Boardwalk, which juts out into the pond. After another long, straight stretch, the trail bends left, putting the visitor-information station and the Yellow Rail Prairie on your right. The yellow rail is one of the most difficult birds to actually see in North America, due to its preference for wet prairies and shallow marshes where bird-watchers rarely go. It is classified as Yellow on the National Audubon Society's WatchList, meaning its numbers are declining but at a slower rate than species in the Red category. At an intersection, go straight and follow the trail as it curves right and reverses direction. Walk past a stand of willows and a small pond.

Continue on the trail toward the visitor-information station and past a sign describing a woodlot that was created to shelter and feed migratory birds. The visitor-information station is now on your left as you approach the entrance road. At the entrance road, turn left to head back to your car. Turning right will take you to a boat launch and East Bay, but the distance makes it best to drive.

■ TO THE TRAILHEAD

From Beltway 8 and I-10, head east 31 miles on I-10 to Exit 812 (TX 61). Go south on TX 61 for 4 miles to a stop sign. Continue through the stop sign as TX 61 becomes TX 562. Go another 8.5 miles to a fork. Bear left on FM 1985 and go 4 miles to the entrance of the refuge, on the right. The visitor-information station is 3 miles ahead.

■ MORE FUN

Other attractions in the area include the **Goose Creek Stream Greenbelt** in Baytown, the **Baytown Nature Center, Eddie V. Gray Wetlands Education and Recreation Center, San Jacinto Point Recreation Area** (**baytown.org/ parks** for more information on all previous), **San Jacinto Battleground State Historic Site** (**tpwd.state.tx.us/spdest/findadest/parks/san_jacinto_ battleground**), the **George and Freda Chandler Arboretum** (**tourismprod .baytown.org/arboretum**), and **Houston Raceway Park** (**houstonraceway .com**). Five miles west of I-10 and TX 61 is the **J. J. Mayes Wildlife Trace** (**www.swg.usace.army.mil/Wallis/Recreation.asp**). East Bay and a boat launch are just minutes south of the preserve entrance.

17 Sam Houston National Forest: Stubblefield North Hike

■ OVERVIEW

LENGTH: 5.7 miles

CONFIGURATION: Out-and-back

SCENERY: Woodlands, creeks, farms

EXPOSURE: Shady

TRAIL TRAFFIC: Light

TRAIL SURFACE: Dirt and grass

HIKING TIME: 3.5 hours

DRIVING DISTANCE: 49 miles from the intersection of Beltway 8 and I-45

ACCESS: Free

MAPS: USGS Moore Grove and San Jacinto; trail maps available at lshtclub.com/mapspage.htm

WHEELCHAIR ACCESS: No

FACILITIES: Trail markers

SPECIAL COMMENTS: There are no facilities on many trails except for parking; be sure to bring sunscreen, bug repellent, water, and food. Pets must be leashed at all times. Motorized vehicles and bicycles are not allowed on the trails. Wear appropriate footwear and long pants.

MORE INFORMATION: (936) 344-6205, www.fs.fed.us/r8/texas/recreation/sam_houston/samhouston_gen_info

■ SNAPSHOT

Sam Houston National Forest, one of four national forests in Texas, covers more than 163,000 acres and is situated between Huntsville, Conroe, Cleveland, and Richards. The Stubblefield North Hike is part of the 128-mile Lone Star Hiking Trail, which has gained National Recreation Trail recognition. The trail winds through the national forest and consists of three major sections: the 40-mile Lake Conroe section, the Central section, and the Winters Bayou–Tarkington Creek section. The trails were developed and are maintained by the Lone Star Hiking Trail Club.

■ UP CLOSE

Head toward the HIKER TRAIL sign and enter the woods. You will be on the Lone Star Hiking Trail, distinguished by silver markers, for the entire hike. The markers are 6–7 feet high in the trees; if you haven't seen a marker in a few minutes, stop and get your

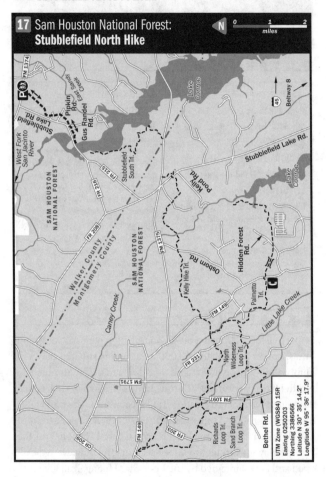

17 Sam Houston National Forest:
Stubblefield North Hike

N 0   1   2
miles

bearings. Look ahead and to both sides, and you should be able to see a marker in the distance. This is a very densely wooded, narrow trail with thick vegetation growing close to the trail surface.

Follow the trail downhill, through several fallen trees. Traverse a rolling section with poor footing (you'll need appropriate footwear for this hike). Go past Trail Marker 26 on the right and an *M* marker in a tree on the left. Hike into and out of a creek bed over exposed tree roots, exposed by washouts. Pass a marker on a tree on the right as the trail narrows again and the foliage encroaches. Wear long pants to prevent exposure to poison ivy. The trail bends right and heads downhill for several hundred yards. Watch for spiderwebs stretching across the trail from early spring to late fall. While the spiders are not poisonous, the webs are a nuisance.

Watch for a trail marker in a tree on the right, and follow the trail as it goes to the right and under a canopy of trees. Go left, following a trail marker in a tree on the right. Although the foliage encroaches, the trail is still easy to see as it heads gradually uphill for a long, straight section. Now descend to a creek bed and hike through it. Climb the other side, hiking over exposed roots.

At an intersection, bear left and hike past a trail marker in a tree on the left. Pass a post with the number 22 on it. Cross a creek bed and climb slightly right on the other side. The trail rises steeply over roots and then goes more moderately uphill. Hike past the "bearing tree" (which helps you find your bearings while hiking) on the right and a national-forest boundary line on a tree on the right. A large stand of young pines comes into view on the right, past an open grassy area. Hike past a hunting blind on your right and head toward a fence. Stay to the left of the fence as the trail bends left. Continue past Trail Marker 22 and a letter *M* in a tree on the right. A small creek is on your right, with the trail going under a canopy of trees and around a large pine tree. Descend into a creek bed and cross it, putting the creek on your left.

Cross another creek bed, then hike uphill and to the right. The trail swings left, with the creek on your left. This is a very winding section of the hike, but numerous trail markers keep you on track. Cross an old road and head back into the trees on the other side, following the trail to the right. The trail then veers left into a creek bed. Across the creek bed, the forest is dark and shady. Make your way over the branches and limbs of a fallen tree, and then climb into and out of another creek bed. Hike through another fallen tree, following the trail as it stretches out ahead of you. Walk over another fallen tree, cross another creek bed, and hike beneath a very large pine tree that has fallen to the other side of the creek. Take a quick right and then a quick left to get back on the trail, which soon heads gradually uphill.

Step through a large cut tree and continue uphill on the grassy trail. Cross a paved road and then, at an intersection, go straight to stay on the trail as it heads uphill, past a deep creek bed on your left. The trail then goes steeply downhill and crosses yet another creek bed, into a dark, shaded area. At an intersection marked by double trail markers on a tree to your left, go right and uphill. At a HIKER TRAIL sign, cross the telephone easement toward the other HIKER TRAIL sign. Pass Trail Marker 21 and an *M* marker in a tree on the left, following the trail downhill. Now hike through an open area with fan palms and oak trees, beyond which the trail narrows to only about a foot wide with many exposed roots and ruts. At the double trail markers on a post on the left, bear right. Hike past the motorized-vehicle barriers and the HIKER TRAIL sign to the road. Turn around and retrace your route to the parking area.

■ TO THE TRAILHEAD

From the intersection of Beltway 8 and I-45, head north 41.5 miles on I-45 and exit at FM 1375/1374. Continue on the feeder road to FM 1374 and turn left, driving over I-45. Drive 7 miles to the trailhead on the left. Look for a very small HIKER TRAIL sign just past the sign for Sam Houston National Forest on the left. Park beside the road in the grass.

■ MORE FUN

Nearby attractions include the **Sam Houston Memorial Museum** (**samhouston.org**), the **Texas Prison Museum** (**txprisonmuseum.org**), the **H.E.A.R.T.S. Veterans Museum** (**heartsmuseum.com**), **Sam Houston National Forest**, and **Lake Conroe**.

Lake Jackson Wilderness Park Trail

■ OVERVIEW

LENGTH: 2 miles

CONFIGURATION: Out-and-back

SCENERY: Bayou, woodlands, bottomland forest

EXPOSURE: Shady with some sun

TRAIL TRAFFIC: Light

TRAIL SURFACE: Grass and dirt

HIKING TIME: 1.5 hours

DRIVING DISTANCE: 39.5 miles from the intersection of Beltway 8 and I-288

ACCESS: Free; open daily, 6 a.m.–10 p.m.

MAPS: USGS Lake Jackson

WHEELCHAIR ACCESS: No

FACILITIES: Parking, picnic areas, fishing, boat ramp

SPECIAL COMMENTS: This is a very small park that is used mainly for hiking and launching small boats, kayaks, or canoes. Primitive camping is allowed with approval. Biking is permitted on the trails, so stay to the right at all times. Do not veer off onto any of the small paths that take you into the forest—these are not part of the park's trail system.

MORE INFORMATION: (979) 297-4533

■ SNAPSHOT

Lake Jackson Wilderness Park is bordered by Buffalo Camp Bayou and the Brazos River bottomland forest. It parallels The Wilderness Golf Course, which you can see a bit of during the hike. Other activities include biking, boating, fishing, picnicking, and bird-watching; there is also an interpretive nature loop. The Gulf Coast Bird Observatory is just across the bayou from the park entrance.

■ UP CLOSE

Start the hike in the parking lot, just to the right of the boat ramp. There are picnic tables and good views of Buffalo Camp Bayou. Continue into the trees past the trail sign and through the gate. The trailhead sign, to the right of the trail, lists the various hikes in the park. As you venture into the trees, the bayou is on your left and the forest is on your right. The wide dirt

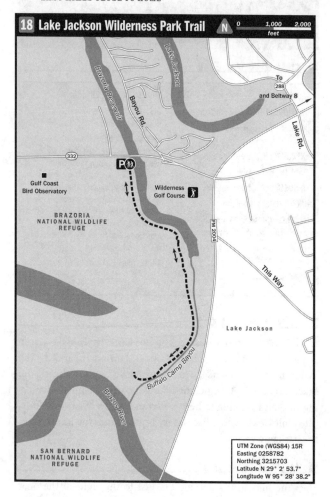

18 Lake Jackson Wilderness Park Trail

N   0   1,000   2,000
feet

To
(288)
and Beltway 8

Lake Rd.

Lake Jackson

Bayou Rd.

Brazoria Reservoir

(332)

Gulf Coast
Bird Observatory

Wilderness
Golf Course

BRAZORIA
NATIONAL WILDLIFE
REFUGE

FM 2004

This Way

Lake Jackson

Buffalo Camp Bayou

Brazos River

SAN BERNARD
NATIONAL WILDLIFE
REFUGE

UTM Zone (WGS84) 15R
Easting 0258782
Northing 3215703
Latitude N 29° 2' 53.7"
Longitude W 95° 28' 38.2"

trail winds through the trees, following the path of the bayou.
Go past a trail marker on the right and continue as the trail
takes a big bend to the left. Stay out of the water and away from
the banks of the bayou, as alligators and poisonous snakes exist

along all the bayous in this part of Texas. As the trail bends right, the trail surface changes to grass; however, it is still easy to follow because it was carved out of the forest. Look to your left across the bayou for the Gulf Coast Bird Observatory headquarters. It has a large picnic pavilion and a small fishing pier, along with nature trails and picnic sites.

Following the trail over a drainage pipe, look to your right to get a brief glimpse of The Wilderness Golf Course. The vegetation on the right is very thick and impenetrable; the foliage on the left can be thick enough in some areas to obscure views of the bayou. The trail narrows and gets even grassier. Go by a 0.25-mile marker on the right. Buffalo Camp Bayou is very wide and the water can run swiftly after heavy rains, so stay on the trail at all times. While hiking, you may see kayakers and canoeists on the bayou. Also look for neotropical migrant birds, such as warblers and wood ducks. Besides alligators, wild pigs are also found in the area, as evidenced by the tracks on the trail. Common plants are sawtooth palmettos, moss-draped oaks, and fan palms.

Continue uphill and to the right, past some large oak trees covered in moss. The trail then heads left, taking you briefly away from the bayou. At a fork, bear left to view the concrete spillway for the bayou. Turn around, head back to the fork, and then head sharply left to get back on the main route. The bayou is still on your left, but it is farther away and you can only see the banks, not the water. The trail swings right, past some low spots; hike around them if they are too wet or muddy to get through. Watch for cyclists at all times, and stay to the right.

The trail winds through the trees and then past a large stand of fan palms on the right. Although the trail surface is grass, it looks like an old road with parallel ruts on each side. Continue as the trail bends right and downhill, over a drainage pipe, and then to the left and uphill. You can hear the traffic on the highway to your left. Once up the hill, the trail swings right. The bayou is still on your left but is not visible. The trail heads uphill out of the trees and into a sunny opening between the vegetation on the right and the bayou on the left. Pass a large oak tree on your left. The bayou is directly on your left now, with the road just to the left of the bayou. You are hiking on the bank of the bayou in an opening that is not a well-defined part of the trail. The route is still easy to follow—just stay between the vegetation on the right and the bayou on the left. Continue as the trail heads downhill off the embankment and then back uphill on the other side.

Look to your right to see how the trees grow in twisted, knotty fashion. They are works of art created by the prevailing winds of the Gulf Coast. Follow the trail as it veers right into the trees, away from the bayou, and then left through a wide, well-defined opening in the forest. Thick foliage is on both sides, with the bayou farther on your left. At a fork, bear left toward the bayou. Now veer right as you pass a trail marker on the right. At a large oak tree on your left, the trail bends to the right, back into the trees. Up ahead you can see the remnants of an old bridge. Turn around and retrace your route to complete the hike.

■ TO THE TRAILHEAD

From Beltway 8 and I-288, head south 38 miles to FM 2004 and take a right. Go 1.3 miles to FM 332 and turn right. The entrance to the park is on the left, just after you cross Buffalo Camp Bayou.

■ MORE FUN

Brazoria National Wildlife Refuge (page 71), the Gulf Coast Bird Observatory (gcbo.org), and San Bernard National Wildlife Refuge (fws.gov/refuges) are less than 15 miles from Lake Jackson Wilderness Park. Brazos Bend State Park (page 52) and George Ranch Historical Park (georgeranch.org), a living-history site and working cattle ranch, are also close by.